Beyond Better:

Thrive

The Carrera Method™

How to Take Control of Your Health, Unlock Your Longevity Genes, and Transform Your Future

Dr. Danielle Carrera, DNP, APRN

Founder, Carrera Telehealth & Wellness

Carrera Telehealth & Wellness

Printed in the United States of America

ISBN 979-8-9939517-2-0

Acknowledgements

This book would not exist without the patients who trusted me with their health, their stories, and their vulnerability. Every person who sat across from me in an exam room — in a long-term care facility, in a clinic in Tampa, through a telehealth screen at all hours of the day or night— taught me something I could not have learned any other way. This book is for them. And because of them.

To my children, Rachel and Chase: you are the reason I built something worth building. Every late night, every sacrifice, every hard decision was made with you in mind. Watching you grow into the people you are becoming is the greatest privilege of my life.

To my husband, Ron: you are my anchor, my partner, and my proof that the right person changes everything. Thank you for choosing me, for cycling with me, and for catching me in all the ways that matter.

To my mother: you showed me what it looks like to walk into the hardest fight of your life with quiet resolve and your head held high. I have been trying to match that courage ever since. Thank you for your great encouragement and love.

To my father: your love is strong, your passion fierce. You set the example of always looking forward to the next great move of your life. It showed me to dream big and to never shrink myself. "Go get 'em baby" is what always stays in my ears and close to my heart.

To my brothers, Dean, Josh, Sal … each with a unique powerful story, each with beautiful families, all three of you warriors, always just a phone call, no matter the time or day… Thank you.

To the team at Carrera Telehealth and Wellness: your commitment to patient-first, judgment-free, evidence-based care makes everything possible. You are not just colleagues. You are proof of what medicine can be.

And to anyone who has ever been told their labs are normal when they knew something was wrong: this book is yours. You were right. Keep asking. Keep advocating. Keep going.

FROM DR. DANIELLE CARRERA DNP, APRN

A Note to the Reader

The information in this book is intended for educational purposes and reflects the clinical experience, perspective, and philosophy of Dr. Danielle Carrera. It is not intended to replace the advice, diagnosis, or treatment provided by a licensed medical professional.

If you are currently under the care of a healthcare provider, please discuss any changes to your health routine — including nutrition, supplementation, hormone therapy, or peptide use — with your provider before making them.

The case studies referenced in this book represent composite or anonymized patient experiences. Identifying details have been changed to protect patient privacy. The clinical principles and outcomes described are reflective of real clinical experience.

Peptides described in this book that carry a Research Use Only (RUO) designation are not FDA-approved for human therapeutic use. Their inclusion is for educational purposes only. Use of RUO peptides should only occur under the direct supervision of a licensed medical provider with appropriate clinical training.

The Carrera Method™ is a framework for integrative wellness education. It is not a diagnostic protocol and does not constitute a clinical treatment plan. Results described in this book are not guaranteed and will vary based on individual circumstances, health history, and adherence.

— Dr. Danielle Carrera, DNP, APRN

Tampa Bay, Florida

Table of Contents

INTRODUCTION

A Nation That Is Not Well

The average American is not well. He, she, they — whatever your pronoun — are inflamed, exhausted, under-screened, overstimulated, and drowning in a culture that has normalized dysfunction. You are skipping routine healthcare, ignoring the early warning signs your body is sending you, and telling yourself you are "fine" — right up until you aren't.

We are living in a nation where 72.4 percent of adults are overweight or obese, according to the National Health and Nutrition Examination Survey. Forty percent meet the clinical criteria for obesity. Nine percent have severe obesity. Nearly three out of four adults weigh more than the recommended range for their height. If you put ten of those individuals in a room, the long-term data tells a sobering story: within a decade, one of them will have a heart attack. That risk climbs steeply for anyone carrying central adiposity, hypertension, insulin resistance, or elevated inflammatory markers.

This is not a crisis of willpower. It is a crisis of awareness, agency, and alignment.

Most people still approach their health the same way: wait for a symptom, go to the doctor, get told their labs are "fine" or that "we'll watch it," leave with nothing actionable except a vague instruction to eat better and exercise more, and repeat that transaction for months and years — until something finally breaks. That is not healthcare. That is damage control. That is sick care dressed up as medicine.

And here is the part that most people do not know: BMI alone dramatically underestimates risk. The markers that truly predict long-term outcomes — visceral fat distribution, ApoB, high-sensitivity C-reactive protein, fasting insulin, waist-to-height ratio — are rarely ordered in a standard eleven-minute primary care visit. The system is not designed to find problems before they announce themselves loudly. It is designed to respond to emergencies.

* * *

I say all of this with authority, because I was on the other side of that exam room door for the better part of almost three decades. I was trained in traditional primary care, urgent care, and long-term care as a nurse practitioner and later as a Doctor of Nursing Practice. I worked for some of the largest healthcare organizations in the country. I saw what the system could do — and more importantly, what it could not. I held my bladder through back-to-back appointments. I skipped lunch. I ran on adrenaline and obligation, giving everything I had to my patients while giving almost nothing to myself.

The irony was not lost on me. If my own cup was empty, how was I genuinely serving the people sitting across from me? Mentally, emotionally, and physically depleted, I was participating in the very system I knew was failing both patients and providers alike.

Something had to change.

* * *

Five years ago, longevity medicine was a luxury most Americans associated with Silicon Valley billionaires and elite performance athletes. Today, it is becoming the standard of care for anyone who refuses to let their health be dictated by chance or by a system that was not built with their optimal outcomes in mind. At Carrera Telehealth and Wellness and expanding now into Above Genetics, we do not wait for disease to introduce itself. We intervene early, strategically, and with intention — because the body gives warnings long before it gives diagnoses.

This book, Beyond Better, Thrive, is not a wellness manifesto. It is not a collection of tips or a thirty-day challenge. It is a reclamation. It is a blueprint for every American — and anyone across the globe — who refuses to settle for "average" in a country where average has come to mean sick, tired, inflamed, and overwhelmed.

This is where science meets sovereignty. Where data becomes direction. Where you stop surviving your life and start designing it.

Welcome to the movement. Welcome to Carrera Telehealth and Wellness. We move with you.

PART ONE

The Breakdown

Why "better" is not enough

CHAPTER ONE

The Moment Everything Changed

My name is Dr. Danielle Carrera. I am a Doctor of Nursing Practice — a DNP, and an autonomous Advanced Practice Registered Nurse licensed in multiple states. I founded and run Carrera Telehealth and Wellness, a practice built on the belief that every person deserves to do more than simply not be sick. By every honest measure, I am living the life I was meant to build.

But getting here was not a straight line. It was a long, circuitous route through grief and grit, through systems that inspired me and systems that nearly broke me, through personal losses that clarified everything. To understand where I am, you have to understand where I came from.

* * *

I grew up in Coral Springs, Florida, in what was, for the most part, a good childhood. My parents divorced when I was two, and by the time I was three, my mother had remarried. My weeks were spent with my mom and stepfather. Most weekends, my older brother Dean and I went to our father's house.

My dad had a gift for making every visit feel like an escape. "When you come to my house," he would say, "you act like you are on vacation." And it did feel that way — easy, warm, and unhurried. He was a loving father, present and generous when he wanted to be. But he also had a capacity for disappearance. If something did not serve him, he could simply switch off — weeks would pass, sometimes months, occasionally years — without explanation. I learned early what it means to love someone who contains multitudes, not all of them comfortable.

Still, my foundation was solid. We were rooted in church and youth group, in an extended web of family and friends. My grandparents' house was a constant anchor — pool water, summer laughter, afternoons that seemed to stretch forever.

My values were established early and they held. Life felt ordered and safe.

Until eleventh grade.

* * *

My mother was diagnosed with breast cancer. She did not hesitate. She chose a mastectomy, followed by chemotherapy and radiation, and she walked into treatment with the same quiet resolve that defined everything she did. By the time I entered my senior year of high school, she was deep in the hardest fight of her life, and I was watching from the periphery, trying to make sense of something no seventeen-year-old should have to process alone.

I was already moving toward medicine in high school. I was enrolled in Health Occupation Students of America and completed clinical rotations as part of my coursework. There is something clarifying about walking into a hospital as a student — the smell, the pace, the weight of what happens inside those walls. I felt, even then, that it was somewhere I belonged.

One afternoon during my clinicals, I walked onto the floor and realized my mother had a room there. She had just come out of surgery. I went in, stayed for a few minutes, checked on her, and walked back out to finish my shift. I did not fall apart. I compartmentalized — filed it somewhere deep and kept moving. That is what I did with all of it, for months. I watched my mother lose her hair. I watched her come home exhausted and nauseous, pull off her wig, and throw it across the room because the heat was unbearable. I absorbed every bit of it quietly, the way I was already learning to absorb hard things.

The moment I finally broke open came in church. I had slept over at my friend's house the night before and arrived a few minutes late, sliding into a row near the back. Four rows ahead, I spotted a woman sitting very still, her back straight, her head completely bare. No wig. No scarf. She had simply decided, on that particular Sunday morning, to show up exactly as she was.

It was my mother.

Something inside me gave way. She looked small in a way I had never allowed myself to see before. She looked like herself and like someone I did not fully recognize. I had been holding my breath for nearly a year without realizing it, and in that moment, looking at the back of her bare head in that quiet church, I finally exhaled. She was still here. She had made it. And somewhere in the white space between that realization and the one that preceded it — that I could have lost her — I cried. Truly cried, for the first time since her diagnosis.

Not in the hospital. Not during a hard conversation. In church, four rows behind my mother on a Sunday morning, I let myself feel how terrified I had been, and how profoundly grateful I was that the fear was behind us.

That experience did not just shape me emotionally. It clarified the direction I was already moving in. Medicine was not simply a career path. It was a calling.

* * *

After graduation, I left Coral Springs and moved to Tampa to attend the University of South Florida. I went alone.

Around the time I enrolled, my mother and stepfather divorced — the aftermath of everything she had been through had taken its toll on the marriage. My father was building his life with his wife and their new family. There was no safety net, no one to call if things fell apart. I understood this clearly, and without self-pity. I was going to have to make it on my own.

I worked multiple jobs and carried a full course load simultaneously. I ended up obtaining my bachelor's degree in psychology. One of my jobs was at Tampa General's Psychiatric Center, where I worked with high-risk adolescent females and court-referred teenage boys in a residential boot camp program. The kids ranged from twelve to nineteen years old. I was twenty-one, twenty-two, twenty-three — barely older than some of them, watching up close what becomes of a child who grows up without a support system. When your environment has failed you comprehensively and from the beginning, the results show up early.

I stayed in that role for about three years, working across the acute, geriatric, and juvenile psychiatric units. I saw Baker

Acts. I saw what a crisis looks like when there is nothing and no one to catch you. It was heavy work, and it mattered.

But I wanted something more clinical. I wanted to be at the bedside, hands-on, inside the full complexity of patient care. So I went back to school to become a registered nurse.

The years that followed — seven or eight years of bedside nursing across med-surg, mother-baby, the PACU, pre-op, and the surgical floor — became the foundation on which everything else was eventually built. I was absorbing every experience, every patient, every outcome. I did not know it yet, but I was in the process of becoming exactly the clinician I was meant to be.

In the middle of all of it, I got married, had two children — my daughter Rachel and my son Chase, who are, without qualification, everything to me — and then navigated a divorce that left me a single mother of a two-and-a-half-year-old and a five-year-old, continuing to work full-time in a demanding field.

Hard times make hard people. I had heard that my whole life. Standing in the middle of everything I was moving into my late twenties and early thirties, I understood it in my bones.

I was being built. I just did not know yet what I was being built for.

CHAPTER TWO

Inside the System

My mother's illness transformed me in ways I did not fully recognize at the time. What I knew was this: I wanted to help people. I wanted to make a genuine difference in their lives, not just a clinical one. I was young, and I believed — the way the young tend to believe before experiencing tempers idealism — that the system would make space for that kind of care. That if you were skilled, dedicated, and compassionate, medicine would meet you there.

As a registered nurse, I was exposed to every corner of the field. I worked alongside physicians, MDs and DOs, nurse practitioners, and physician assistants. I assisted anesthesiologists. I helped transfer patients off helicopters and into the emergency department. I saw the full spectrum of acute care, from the mundane to the extraordinary, and I loved nearly all of it.

But I also started noticing the architecture of the system itself — and the ways it worked against the care I wanted to provide. Everything had a clock on it. Every interaction was bounded by time constraints, billing codes, and throughput metrics. I understood that healthcare is a business with real financial pressures. What I did not understand yet was how thoroughly those pressures had come to override clinical judgment. Nurses were the right hand of every upper-level provider in that building. We were essential. And none of us had enough time to give patients what they fundamentally needed.

I watched things get missed. Patients would come in after traumatic events — multiple fractures, head injuries, lacerations requiring sutures or staples — and in the churn of a busy floor, details would fall through. Staples were never documented. No one followed up on their removal. Patients were discharged into inadequate situations, with no family to help them and no plan beyond "follow up with your doctor."

I kept returning to the same thought: I can do more than this. There has to be a better way to practice.

* * *

After my divorce, with a two-and-a-half-year-old and a five-year-old at home, I applied to the University of South Florida's nurse practitioner program. There were four hundred applicants for seventeen seats. The program required more than academic credentials — three letters of professional reference, two formal papers, and multiple rounds of interviews, each piece weighted and evaluated carefully. It was rigorous, as it should have been.

My grades were strong and my references were solid. It all came down to the interviews. By the final round, I had answered the same fundamental questions several times: Why this program? What would you contribute? What makes you different? I had run out of polished answers. So when the interviewer asked one more time, I said simply, "Because I'm a good egg." He laughed. I laughed. And I received my acceptance letter.

I called my mother first. Her response was characteristically measured: "Well… now what are you going to do?" She was not wrong to ask. I lived four hours from the nearest family member. My children's father was not involved. I was going to have to work full-time, complete full-time clinical residencies, and raise two small children simultaneously. What I told her — what I told myself — was the only honest answer available: "I don't know, but I'll make it work."

There was no celebration. No one said they were proud of me. I do not think people outside of medicine fully understand what it costs to do this work at this level — the years of education, the financial burden, the personal sacrifices that never make it into any job description. Anyone who chooses this profession and sees it through deserves to be recognized for that.

I studied from early morning until late at night, getting up only when necessary to use the bathroom and make a frozen meal. I hired babysitters and relied on friends to help with childcare. I did not go to the beach on weekends. While my friends were living the lives of people in their twenties, I was in a small home office surrounded by textbooks, building something I could not yet fully see.

* * *

My first clinical rotation was in neurosurgery at Tampa General Hospital — a rotation I should not have been scheduled for until the end of the nurse practitioner program, but which I received early by default as there were no other clinical rotations open. To say the least, it was extraordinary. The complexity of neurological care, the precision required, the stakes involved — it engaged every part of my clinical mind in a way nothing had before. It set the foundation for my responsibility that someone's life and care can begin and end with me and me only.

I also rotated through a rural clinic where a physician treated patients without insurance at deeply reduced cost. The contrast with the hospital system was immediate and instructive. I saw construction workers come in with metal shavings embedded in their corneas — injuries that, in a hospital setting, would have been referred to ophthalmology.

In this clinic, we numbed the eye, used specialized scopes, and removed the fragments ourselves with bent sterile needles. We worked with what we had.

The clinical details mattered. I learned that if metal remains in the eye for more than four to six hours, a rust ring can form, and tetanus prophylaxis becomes necessary. In small clinics without robust protocols, those details were often missed. In hospitals, there were systems for everything. The disparity in outcomes was not abstract to me — I was watching it happen in real time.

What I also began seeing clearly was the weight that the system placed on its providers. The number of patients. The administrative burden. The emotional load of work that is, by its nature, never finished. Providers were doing remarkable things inside an infrastructure that was grinding them down. The system was not designed to sustain the people running it. And something, I was certain, was fundamentally missing.

CHAPTER THREE

The Education Gap

One of my earliest positions as a nurse practitioner was performing fit-for-duty physicals for firefighters and law enforcement officers. It was a government-supported prevention program — and rightfully so. Firefighters are occupationally exposed to carcinogens on a scale most people do not appreciate. The cancers that follow — thyroid, testicular, renal, and others — are well-documented. These programs existed to catch problems early, before they became irreversible.

What I was not fully prepared for was the degree of systemic dysfunction I would find in people who were otherwise considered healthy enough to do physically demanding work. Their sleep patterns were severely disrupted — circadian rhythms completely dysregulated by shift work. And when circadian rhythm breaks down, it cascades: cognitive function suffers, metabolic rate changes, cellular repair slows. I believe, and the emerging research supports, that this kind of chronic disruption is one of the mechanisms that activates cancer-related gene expression in susceptible individuals.

These were people in physically demanding careers, expected to be strong and capable, who were quietly falling apart from the inside. Their testosterone levels were suppressed. Their energy was gone in ways that exceeded normal fatigue. Their hormones were not functioning. And because they were presented as "fine" by conventional standards, no one had looked closely enough to see what was in fact happening.

We performed comprehensive evaluations: organ ultrasounds, cardiovascular stress tests, echocardiograms, extensive laboratory panels, hearing assessments, and vision testing. The findings were consistent and sobering. Law enforcement officers with significant sensorineural hearing loss. Firefighters with uncontrolled asthma and chronic upper-respiratory disease. And always, the looming shadow of cancer risk that these individuals carried as an occupational constant.

These programs saved lives — of that I have no doubt. They identified conditions that would have otherwise remained invisible until they became emergencies. It was the kind of proactive, prevention-focused medicine I believed in deeply. And it reinforced what I was beginning to understand as a foundational principle: the body gives warnings long before it gives diagnoses.

* * *

My next position shifted the landscape entirely. I took a job in an underserved area of Tampa to qualify for a federal loan repayment program — nearly a year of service in exchange for $75,000 in tax-free student loan reimbursement. The salary was lower than I was worth, and I accepted that trade deliberately. I wanted the clinical experience more than I wanted the income.

What I got was the most concentrated medical education of my career.

The clinic was staffed by two physicians, four nurse practitioners, and two physician assistants. We were busy every day without exception. Each of us was expected to see approximately twenty-five patients daily, and the patient population represented a cross-section of humanity that no residency program could have prepared me for.

We saw incarcerated individuals requiring pre-release physicals. Women engaged in sex work who came in weekly for treatment. Undocumented immigrants who were terrified to seek care anywhere else. Patients from the opposite end of the social spectrum — high-income individuals who did not want to be recognized in the traditional healthcare system. Many tested positive for syphilis, HIV, chlamydia, and gonorrhea. I had patients go into active myocardial infarction in my exam room and had to call 911.

Most of these individuals had no established care. They came to us only when something had progressed beyond what they could ignore. I've had patients walk through my doors in full diabetic ketoacidosis — breathing in that deep, labored Kussmaul pattern, carrying the unmistakable sweet acetone scent on their breath, and with blood sugars so high they couldn't even register on a standard glucometer — completely unaware they had diabetes until that very moment. Medical emergencies were not occasional. They were the rhythm of the day.

I treated homeless patients who had been living without basic sanitation for extended periods. I saw young men — seventeen, eighteen years old — coming in for their first employment physicals with hygiene so severely neglected that I had to send them back to their shelter to bathe before I could complete the visit. No one had ever taught them. Not because they were unintelligent, but because no one in their lives had ever had the occasion to. I found myself explaining, in a clinical setting, how to wash clothing, apply antibacterial soap, and use antiperspirant — because I was the first person who had ever told them.

People are products of their environment. This is not a controversial statement. It is a clinical reality. And many of the patients I saw in that clinic had been produced by environments that had failed them from the beginning.

* * *

I used every minute of those eleven-minute appointments. I was direct, sometimes bluntly so — because I would rather a patient feel momentarily embarrassed in my exam room than publicly humiliated at a job interview or in a social situation. Hygiene, dental health, sexual health, nutrition — nothing was off limits. I was not there to make people comfortable. I was there to give them information they could use.

And yet, even my most direct interventions ran into the walls that the system had built around these patients. Medications that cost six or seven dollars were refused. Visits offered at no cost or at twenty-five dollars were still met with resistance from patients who had been conditioned by the system to expect everything to be provided without charge. The entitlement was not malicious — it was institutional. They had been taught, by years of experience, that healthcare was something that happened to them rather than something they participated in.

That was when the realization crystallized for me. The system is broken — yes. Government policy has failed these communities — yes. But at a certain point, individual responsibility must also be part of the conversation. The capacity to change the course of one's health exists in every person. What is often missing is someone willing to tell the truth about what it requires.

I did not know it at the time, but that clinic — loud, exhausting, and unlike anything I had ever experienced — was where the philosophy that would anchor my entire career began to take shape.

Be the CEO of your own health.

That idea was not born in a seminar or a business plan. It was born in an eleven-minute appointment in the roughest clinic in Tampa, where I learned that the most powerful intervention a provider can offer is not a prescription — it is information, delivered with enough honesty and enough care to change how someone sees themselves in relation to their own body.

PART TWO

The Awakening

Discovering there is a *better* way

CHAPTER FOUR

The Practitioner Who Started Asking Why

I lasted just under a year in that clinic. The hours were not sustainable, and more importantly, they were costing me time with my children that I could not get back. Rachel and Chase were young. The window for being genuinely present in their lives was finite, and I was spending it in an environment that consumed everything I had. I needed to recalibrate.

I started, as clinicians often do, with my own family. I made sure my children's preventive care was current — dental cleanings, well-child visits, the baseline screenings that matter more than most parents realize. And I turned that same attention on myself. I checked my own laboratory values. My vitamin D was significantly deficient. I was not anemic, but I was not optimized. I had been so focused on taking care of everyone else that I had effectively neglected the most basic aspects of my own health. It was a humbling realization for someone who spent her professional life telling patients to do better.

I joined UnitedHealthcare, one of the largest managed care organizations in the country. On paper, it looked like an upgrade: a salary with performance bonuses, a defined patient panel, and a role that promised structure after years of clinical chaos.

What it fundamentally delivered was one of the most rigorous clinical educations of my career.

* * *

My patients at UnitedHealthcare were the sickest of the sick — individuals with multiple comorbidities, managing five, eight, ten chronic conditions simultaneously, on medication lists so long they required their own document. To care for them well, I had to become fluent in specialties I had never formally received extensive training in. I read pulmonology literature and took advanced continuing education for several months on a Tuesday, nephrology on a Thursday, neurology on the weekend. Diabetes and medication management was second nature to me, and I felt extremely competent until my dementia patient decided today was the day they were not going to eat at all, refusing even fluids after being given their morning insulin. The nurses and I learned real fast no routine scheduled humalog or novolog until the patient was three fourths deep into their meal. I studied and became very familiar with antibiotics and out of the norm diseases that arose with severely immunocompromised patients, how to treat them and what medication was priority. I also continuously consulted with specialty providers and absorbed their reasoning for their treatment regimen. Skin infections and wounds that refused to heal was a daily battle. So many times rashes that you thought they were finally gone came back with a vengeance. I ordered stat labs, chest X-rays, midlines, breathing treatments, and IV antibiotics, all while monitoring for acute changes and silently hoping the nurses' station wouldn't call with an emergent decline. In that pressure cooker, I learned to synthesize complex, competing clinical priorities and make decisions that held patients together long enough to keep them stable. The model was designed around outcomes: bonuses tied to A1C control, cholesterol targets, blood pressure management, and hospital avoidance. In principle, it aligned financial incentives with patient health. In practice, it was more complicated. The pressure to keep patients out of the hospital sometimes created tension with the clinical judgment that said a patient needed to be in one. I held my ground. When someone fell and hit their head, when vitals were unstable, when the presentation was ambiguous in a way that made me uncomfortable — I sent them to the hospital. My license and my moral compass were never negotiable.

But the ethical pressure escalated over time. Diagnosis coding practices began to shift toward the highest-acuity codes allowable under Medicare guidelines, regardless of whether the clinical picture fully supported them. The incentive was financial, tied to risk-adjustment formulas that rewarded documented complexity. I understood the mechanism. I was not comfortable with the application. That discomfort was a signal I filed away and returned to later.

* * *

The position did offer one significant benefit: continuing medical education. I attended conferences regularly, which is how I found myself in Orlando in October of 2019, rotating through a pharmaceutical exhibition floor where representatives were showcasing new and emerging medications.

Three stopped me.

The first was a treatment for basal cell carcinoma — a targeted oral agent that could slow or halt the proliferation of cancerous cells in elderly patients who were not surgical candidates. The clinical implications were significant. The price point, at $11,000 per month, was disqualifying for most patients without comprehensive insurance.

The second was an advanced inhaler combination for COPD and asthma — technically impressive, clinically meaningful for the right patient population.

The third changed the direction of my career.

It was a GLP-1 receptor agonist called Trulicity, developed by Eli Lilly. The mechanism was elegant: a once-weekly subcutaneous injection that stimulated insulin secretion only in the presence of food, dramatically reducing the risk of hypoglycemia that had made so many patients fearful of injectable diabetes medications. It was not insulin. It was a peptide — a class of compounds I was about to become deeply acquainted with.

The clinical profile was exactly what my patients needed: lower A1Cs, reduced hypoglycemic events, decreased polypharmacy, less nursing burden from daily injections and finger sticks, cardiovascular protection, and — significantly — meaningful weight loss in patients who were largely sedentary and had been unable to lose weight through conventional means. For the older adults in long-term care facilities I was managing, this was transformative.

I began prescribing Trulicity widely. The results were unambiguous. Nurses noticed. Other providers noticed. Colleagues started calling me to ask what I was doing differently. I began explaining, informally at first, and then with increasing structure.

Eli Lilly noticed too. My prescribing numbers appeared in their national data, and their pharmaceutical representative — a remarkable woman named, Lourdes who had been assigned to my territory and who becamea genuine colleague and friend — connected me with the regional medical director/manager. They asked if I would become a national provider speaker for Trulicity.

Teaching has always been intrinsic to how I practice. I had spent nearly four years instructing LPN and RN students during my NP schooling at Jersey College of Nursing as an instructor, and I had precepted nurse practitioner students throughout my career as an APRN . Stepping into a formal education role for a pharmaceutical company felt like a natural extension of something I already did. I accepted.

I traveled to long-term care facilities, rehabilitation centers, and primary care practices across the region, teaching providers about GLP-1 pharmacology, patient selection, and the outcomes data that were beginning to accumulate. I learned more about diabetes management and the emerging science of metabolic medicine during that period than in any single clinical role before it. The feedback from my patients was consistent and deeply gratifying: better laboratory values, fewer medications, weight loss that had felt impossible for years, and a quality of life that had meaningfully improved.

This was where the transformation truly began — the first moment I understood that the tools available in medicine were expanding in ways that the standard of care had not yet caught up to.

CHAPTER FIVE

What I Saw Behind the Curtain of Corporate Medicine - The Part No One Talks About

---

Seven years is long enough to understand a system from the inside. Long enough to see its architecture clearly — what it was designed to do, what it was never designed to do, and what it actively prevented.

UnitedHealthcare taught me discipline. It taught me to listen with the kind of attention that produces real clinical insight — not just to what patients said, but to what they could not articulate, to what the family in the corner of the room was afraid to ask, to what the nursing notes suggested between the lines. It taught me to think in systems, to follow a patient through multiple transitions of care and hold the thread of their history without losing a single relevant detail. Continuity of care was not a concept I practiced in that role. It was the entire job.

Those years also showed me, with increasing clarity, where the system ended and where better medicine had to begin.

* * *

The model was structured around outcomes metrics: hospital admission rates, A1C control, blood pressure targets, medication adherence scores. UnitedHealthcare's stated goal was to keep patients out of the hospital. My goal was to keep them alive — and those two objectives were not always the same thing. When they diverged, I chose my patients. Every time. My moral compass was not a professional liability. It was my most important clinical tool.

But the structural pressures were real and they escalated over time. Patient panels grew larger. Geographic territories expanded. Providers were driving hours between visits, juggling administrative demands that multiplied annually, and absorbing the emotional weight of managing individuals with catastrophic, irreversible disease — all while being evaluated primarily on metrics that told an incomplete story about the quality of care being delivered.

The most troubling pressure was the one I have already referenced: the incentive to code diagnoses at the highest clinically defensible level to maximize risk-adjustment reimbursement from Medicare. I understood the financial logic. I was not comfortable with the clinical ethics. There is a meaningful difference between accurate, thorough documentation and systematically inflating acuity. I drew that line and I held it.

* * *

COVID revealed everything.

Four months prior to COVID I decided to start my own little Telehealth practice more for compliance when family or friends asked for a prescription for a sinus infection or traditional medication refills. I needed a place to land my documentation and stay in compliance with the board of nursing / medicine. It also felt great to have my own little practice. I had no idea how this was setting the foundation and the roots for what was about to come fast and furious in the next few months.

When the pandemic arrived, it did not create new problems in the healthcare system. It exposed the ones that had been there all along. The infrastructure collapsed under pressure it was never engineered to withstand. Patients could not access their primary care providers. They could not get refills for medications they had been taking for years. People with serious respiratory illness sat at home without guidance because every clinic and hospital was overwhelmed or closed to non-emergencies. The system that was supposed to catch people had no safety net built into it for exactly this kind of moment.

My telehealth practice — which I had been building alongside my employed position for the last several months — became something patients needed urgently. It was not a side project anymore. It was a refuge. A place where the practice of medicine could continue to be responsive, human, and individualized, even when everything around it was collapsing. I partnered with a physician in my everyday job at UHC who believed in clinical autonomy and patient-first decision-making. He embraced regenerative medicine and holistic medicine and embraced new approaches such as ivermectin to shorten the duration of the COVID virus and the intensity. Because he was my collaborating physician for so many years and was in his own autonomous practice, not corporation bound with system protocols, he could think outside the box. UHC allowed me to follow his protocol with ivermectin. We did what the system could not. We treated the patient to the best of our ability without doing harm but only for the ultimate good.

That experience made one thing irreversible: I could no longer participate in a model that rewarded compliance over clinical judgment. I had seen, clearly and finally, what medicine looked like when it was allowed to be practiced the way it should be — and I could not unsee it.

The truth about large healthcare organizations is not complicated. They are engineered to keep providers productive enough to be valuable and exhausted enough not to leave. It is a system that depends on a particular kind of depletion — one that is gradual enough to be tolerable but sustained enough to be disabling. I felt that pull. I felt the burnout accumulating. And I felt, simultaneously and with increasing urgency, something stronger than any of it: the certainty that I was built to do something different.

I did not want autonomy for the sake of independence. I wanted it for the sake of what I could do with it.

That conviction became the turning point. Not a dramatic resignation or a single defining moment — just the quiet, firm decision that I was done practicing inside walls that were too small for the kind of medicine I knew was possible.

CHAPTER SIX

The World of Peptides and Possibility

My serious introduction to peptide-based medicine began, as so many pivotal clinical moments do, in an unlikely setting: a continuing medical education conference in Orlando, rotating through pharmaceutical exhibition tables with a group of colleagues, earning the required signatures to maintain my licensure.

I stopped at the Eli Lilly booth. What the representative placed in front of me was a once-weekly injectable GLP-1 receptor agonist called Trulicity a dulaglutide — a compound I have described in an earlier chapter, but whose significance to this particular story bears revisiting from a different angle. Because what I was encountering at that table was not just a diabetes medication. It was my first real exposure to the therapeutic potential of peptides as a class.

Trulicity is a glucagon-like peptide-1 receptor agonist. GLP-1 is an incretin hormone produced naturally in the gut in response to food intake. It stimulates insulin secretion in a glucose-dependent manner — meaning it only activates when blood sugar is elevated, so when a person eats. If they do not eat it is not activated and the fear of hypoglycemia with regular insulin becomes much less of a concern. This of course was great for my dementia patients who decide at the drop of a hat to abandon all food for the day and go on strike to let anyone check their blood sugar. GLP 1's such as Trulicity suppress glucagon release. It slows gastric emptying which makes them feel fuller and hence not overeat. And, critically, it does all of this with a pharmacological precision that significantly reduces the hypoglycemic risk that has made injectable diabetes therapy so feared by patients and burdensome for nursing staff.

For my patient population — older adults in long-term care facilities, many of them sedentary, managing multiple comorbidities, already on complex medication regimens — this represented a meaningful clinical advance. Fewer finger sticks. Fewer hypoglycemic episodes. Reduced polypharmacy. Measurable cardiovascular protection. And, as an additional and often life-changing effect: weight loss in patients who had been unable to achieve it through any other intervention.

It becomes a clinical causality dilemma: did the patient gain weight because of reduced mobility from the degenerative knee or hip fracture, or did the excess weight itself impair healing and perpetuate functional decline? It didn't matter, my patients were benefiting from it more than any other pharma medication. In an odd way, it was like the fountain of youth giving my patients a second chance to take hold of their life, their health. They could eat and not feel shamed, they felt full and in control, they now had some authority over how many fingersticks they were getting. Their A1C and lipid panels, all their labs benefitted, and people started to notice. It was a win-win. I prescribed it broadly.

The results were unambiguous. That is when Eli Lilly Pharmaceuticals invited me to lunch. Little did I know that day that I would become a national provider speaker for Eli Lilly and for Trulicity. I accepted the role with genuine joy and the kind of conviction that only comes from seeing a therapy transform outcomes in real time. Trulicity — a GLP-1 peptide that mimics a hormone the body naturally produces, this was a true game changer. It offered a physiologic, evidence-based approach that finally moved the needle for patients who had struggled for years.

Stepping into that role felt like the perfect alignment of my clinical experience, my passion for metabolic medicine, and my commitment to bringing forward therapies that work with the body rather than against it. It was not the usual question of "what do we need to do to stop the negative outcome" but more "what can we offer the body to help correct signaling messages, or communication to support its own healing?" What made it even more meaningful was knowing that this wasn't just about my own patients. It was an opportunity to support clinicians across the country who were navigating the same challenges in diabetes care, giving them a tool that could genuinely shift trajectories.

Becoming part of that educational movement became one of the most rewarding extensions of my practice — a chance to advocate for a therapy that was both biologically precise and clinically effective.

* * *

The next chapter of the peptide story arrived with Mounjaro — a tirzepatide, a dual-agonist targeting both the GLP-1 and GIP receptors. GIP, or glucose-dependent insulinotropic polypeptide, is a second incretin hormone with complementary mechanisms. The dual-agonist approach produced glycemic control and weight loss outcomes that surpassed anything in the prior generation of medications. I was invited to be on the board of providers for Eli Lilly's new drug "Mounjaro" and to launch it into long term care. There were only five of us on this board representing all the United States. We were the top clinicians utilizing Trulicity and now Mounjaro. This later led to increasing education and real live and life clinical research. I became an expert in all the "tides "to include dulaglutide, liraglutide, semaglutide, tirzepatide. So, when the FDA approved the new weight loss drug with the dual peptide called Zepbound, the trajectory of my Carrera Telehealth and Wellness practice shifted once again. My

Carrera Telehealth and Wellness medical practice was saturated with patients wanting to utilize these peptides to maximize diabetes control but also do something worldly impossible, loose substantial weight that was otherwise never capable of safely doing. I was so educated in all the research and statistics from being a National Provider Speaker for Eli Lilly that my confidence and competency in prescribing and educating patients far surpassed any providers in my field.

These were not incremental improvements. They were, for many patients, transformative. Individuals who had carried significant excess weight for decades, who had been told by multiple providers over many years that they needed to "eat less and move more," were losing twenty, thirty, fifty, in some cases over a hundred pounds — and maintaining that loss in ways no prior intervention had enabled. The clinical implications extended well beyond aesthetics: metabolic markers improved, inflammatory burden decreased, cardiovascular risk profiles changed, joint pain resolved, sleep apnea remitted.

And then insurance coverage contracted, coupon programs ended, and the patients who had achieved the most dramatic results suddenly faced the prospect of reverting. They were not willing to accept that. And they were determined to find an alternative whether I helped them or not.

* * *

Compounded tirzepatide and semaglutide — versions of these peptides produced by compounding pharmacies during periods of FDA-declared shortage — emerged as the primary alternative for patients who could not access or afford the branded medications. My patients were asking about them. Some had already sourced them independently.

I made a deliberate clinical decision. If my patients were going to pursue compounded peptides — and the evidence suggested they were going to do so regardless of my guidance — then my responsibility was to ensure they did it as safely as possible. I identified a compounding pharmacy operating under strict regulatory oversight, one that provided certificates of analysis for every batch, screened rigorously for endotoxins, and maintained the quality controls necessary to ensure patient safety. I was transparent with my patients about the distinction between compounded and branded formulations. I documented risks. I monitored outcomes.

What I observed over the months that followed pushed me in a direction I had not anticipated.

* * *

It was during my own recovery from a serious pelvic fracture — described in full in the chapter that follows — that I encountered the next layer of peptide medicine. Searching for anything that might accelerate tissue repair and support recovery beyond what standard rehabilitation protocols offered, I began researching BPC-157 and TB-500, the synthetic fragment of thymosin beta-4.

BPC-157, or Body Protective Compound 157, is a synthetic pentadecapeptide derived from a protein found in gastric juice. The preclinical literature on its regenerative properties is extensive in animals — accelerated tendon and ligament healing, improved angiogenesis, modulation of inflammatory pathways, and neuroprotective effects. TB-500 similarly acts through actin-binding mechanisms that promote tissue repair, angiogenesis, and cell migration.

Very few providers were using these compounds in clinical practice. The regulatory landscape was complex — neither peptide held FDA approval for therapeutic use in humans at the time, though they were available through compounding pharmacies for research or clinical application at provider discretion. I approached the evidence as I approached all evidence: with rigor, with appropriate skepticism, and with a clear-eyed acknowledgment of what the data could and could not support.

I dove in. I studied literature systematically. I used both compounds much later in my own recovery. I monitored my response with the same discipline I applied to patient care. And what I observed — both in myself and subsequently in patients for whom I prescribed these agents under careful clinical supervision with education as they are "research use only"- RUO — was consistently and compellingly positive.

The experience reframed how I thought about medicine entirely.

Traditional pharmaceutical medicine, for all its extraordinary accomplishments, operates primarily at the level of symptom suppression and disease management. It asks: What is wrong, and how do we stop it? Peptide-based and regenerative medicine asks a fundamentally different question: What does the body need to repair itself, and how do we provide it? The therapeutic targets are different. The philosophy is different. And for the patients who had been failed by the conventional model, the outcomes were often dramatically different.

This was the moment my career shifted from conventional sick-care to a new frontier: cellular optimization, regenerative healing, and the science of making the body not merely functional, but exceptional.

I was not just prescribing medications anymore. I was building a practice around a different model of what medicine could be. And I was absolutely committed to it.

PART THREE

The Thrive Model

How to take control of your health

CHAPTER SEVEN

The Accident That Forced Alignment

The turning point did not look like a turning point. It arrived on an ordinary Saturday, on a bicycle path in good weather, in the early weeks of a relationship that would become my marriage.

My now-husband and I were cycling together — we were six weeks in, still in that early period of discovering each other, still playful and a little reckless. I reached back to grab the hem of his shirt. A flirtatious, thoughtless gesture. We were cycling quite fast as we had done on previous occasions. But this time, his front pedal caught my front tire. The physics were immediate and unforgiving: I was launched forward, my body connecting with the crossbar and handlebars before the momentum flipped me over the bike entirely, and I landed on my head.

The moment I made contact with the ground; I knew. Twenty-five years of clinical experience translated into a single, immediate assessment: my pelvis was fractured.

I was dry heaving from pain (this is a natural sign when a bone is broken). I was losing consciousness in waves. The pain was not a specific sensation so much as a total systemic event, my body was in shock. An ambulance arrived and the situation escalated quickly to a trauma activation as my BP was 80/40—and the fracture didn't need diagnostic testing to present itself, as it was an open fracture. My shorts were torn, and my left labia had a thick wide laceration. The pelvis is among the most vascular structures in the body, and an open pelvic fracture carries a significant risk of internal hemorrhage. I was rushed via ambulance and soon it was determined I needed surgery. The open fracture required partial resection of the involved bone.

* * *

There is a video of me, taken a few hours after surgery, smiling and laughing. People assume it was the anesthesia or the pain medication. It was not. What I felt in that moment was relief.

Relief is not the word most people would expect from someone who had just fractured her pelvis and undergone emergency surgery. But twenty-five years of working in medicine at the pace and intensity I had maintained had produced something that no single health crisis or warning sign had been able to interrupt: a state of continuous, cumulative exhaustion that I had simply normalized. I had been running on it for so long that I did not recognize it as exhaustion anymore. It was just the baseline.

Lying in that hospital bed, I felt it lift. Something inside me finally exhaled.

The accident forced what no act of will had been able to accomplish: a complete stop. An enforced pause long enough to see the life I had been living from the outside. I had a clarity of vision that I had not experienced in years. I knew, with the certainty that comes from a body that has been pushed past its limits and has finally been given permission to rest, that I was not going back to what I had been doing.

That is a tragic way to arrive at clarity. I know that. I am honest about it. I know myself well enough to acknowledge that if the accident had not happened, I would have pushed through whatever warnings came next. I would have flagged symptoms and deferred treatment. I would have told myself I would deal with it later. I have watched myself do exactly that for two and a half decades. It took a fractured pelvis to make "later" unavoidable.

* * *

Recovery was not graceful. I went home with a walker. I had to relearn how to ambulate, how to navigate stairs, how to perform the most basic acts of daily living without assistance. I attended physical therapy multiple times weekly. I was in pain. I was also, for the first time in my career, in the position my patients occupied — dependent on a healthcare system that I now understood from the inside, as a recipient rather than a provider.

Two days after surgery, I learned that my trauma surgeon had "left the practice". Rumor had it he was inundated and decided his mental health was far more important and he was taking a hiatus from being a trauma surgeon.... Go figure. He was burned out, overwhelmed, finished by the same system I had been trapped in for years.

My follow-up care would be transferred to another physician in the practice. I later discovered that provider had back-to-back patients and I was pushed out to a PA who was competent but felt my sutures weren't ready to come out yet and to follow up in a week. Well... my suture removal appointment for that following week was surprisingly (total sarcasm in my voice right now) rescheduled without notice. I could not wait another 10 days in fear the sutures would bury themselves into my tissue and become infected. I sat with that problem for approximately twenty minutes before I propped a mirror against the wall and removed the sutures myself.

What I was experiencing was not unusual. It was exactly what millions of Americans experience when they need care: fragmented follow-up, providers in transition, logistical barriers that seem small in the abstract but are enormous when you are physically impaired and in pain. The system did not fail me dramatically. It simply did what systems without adequate continuity inevitably do — it provided whatever it could in the moment and left the gaps for the patient to manage.

* * *

I chose not to spend my recovery in resentment. I chose, instead, to use it.

This was still during the height of COVID, and the patients I served through my telehealth practice were in genuine crisis. They could not access their primary care providers. They could not get medication refills. They had no one to answer their questions about symptoms that were frightening them. I worked from home, from the couch, on a walker — and I expanded my practice during what should have been the most personally difficult period of my life, because the need was real and because I could.

I also gave myself, with discipline and intention, what I had spent years giving my patients: time to heal. Not just physically. The accident created the space to examine the beliefs I had been carrying — about medicine, about my role within it, about what I was willing to accept as a permanent way of practicing — and to release the ones that no longer served me. I allowed myself to grieve the years spent in a model that had not been built for the kind of care I wanted to provide. And I opened myself to what was becoming increasingly clear about what I was going to build instead.

I learned something about recovery that I had known intellectually but now understood physiologically: healing is impossible when the body is locked in fight-or-flight. Chronic cortisol elevation sustained sympathetic activation, the physiological architecture of constant vigilance — none of it is compatible with cellular repair. I had to work, actively and deliberately, to shift my nervous system into a state in which healing could truly occur. I used breath work. I practiced emotional processing. I leaned into prayer and the kind of quiet I had not allowed myself in years. I did five-minute gratitude practices two or three times a week, which sounds trivial until you understand what those five minutes really do to the biochemistry of recovery.

Slowly, and then more quickly, I felt safe again.

* * *

The accident that fractured my pelvis rebuilt something more important: the certainty of what I was meant to do next. It became the foundation of my destiny — to teach, to lead, and to stand as living proof of what it means to become the CEO of your own health.

CHAPTER EIGHT

Building a New Model of Care - Freedom was Not Quiet

Freedom, when it finally came, was not quiet. It arrived in full force — loud and immediate and completely aligned with everything I had been moving toward for years.

Once I stepped out of employed medicine and into autonomous practice, the acceleration was almost disorienting. My telehealth platform expanded faster than I had projected. GLP-1 therapies — Mounjaro, Zepbound, Ozempic, Wegovy — were creating a category of clinical results that had never existed before at this scale: patients who had lived with significant obesity for decades were losing weight in ways that were medically meaningful and sustained. The demand was extraordinary. I leaned into it completely. People with Covid and long Covid requested ivermectin and treatment protocols aligned with research from FLCCC like their life dependent on it … because it did.

I hired five nurse practitioners, each selected not only for clinical competence but for philosophical alignment. Patient-first. Judgment-free. Evidence-based. We operated seven days a week, around the clock, because patients in a telehealth model do not have health emergencies on a Monday-through-Friday schedule. Urgent care. Primary care. Weight-loss medicine. Regenerative medicine. The practice became a full ecosystem of care, and it was thriving in a way I had never experienced in an employed position.

My days were long. They were also, for the first time in my career, entirely mine. As my friend Bill Walsh says, "We are the only ones willing to work 100 plus hours, so we do not have to work 40 hours for someone else."

* * *

As the practice expanded, new clinical opportunities opened. I began performing G-physicals at three different academies — neurological-based evaluations required for individuals in high-security environments who carry weapons professionally. This was specialized, high stakes work that required the full depth of my clinical training and the kind of judgment that only comes with years of experience across multiple systems of care. It was also, unexpectedly, one of the more rewarding parts of my practice. I worked with retired law enforcement officers who had stories that filled entire rooms. Military contractors. People making significant career transitions. It was a patient population that was simultaneously rigorous and deeply human.

Life was moving faster than it ever had. And it was aligned in a way it had never previously been. I was not surviving the day anymore. I was not arriving at the end of each week depleted and relieved that it was over. I was building something — deliberately, incrementally, with clear intention and the clinical freedom to execute it — and the building itself was energizing.

The model I was creating reflected everything I had wished the system had been for me during the decades I had worked inside it: accessible, responsive, individualized, and built around the patient's actual needs rather than the constraints of whoever was paying the bill. It was not a novel concept. It was simply medicine practiced the way it is supposed to be practiced, without the institutional layers that had spent years getting in the way.

Freedom looked like growth. Freedom looked like impact. Freedom looked like stepping, finally, into the role I was always meant to hold.

For the first time in my career, life was not simply happening to me. I was directing it.

CHAPTER NINE

Beyond Better—What Thriving Actually Means

Most people believe the opposite of "sick" is "healthy." It is not. The opposite of sick is simply not sick — a neutral, fragile, impermanent state in which symptoms are quiet but the underlying dysfunction is still present. Still accumulating. Still moving in the wrong direction, slowly enough that no one sounds an alarm.

I did not understand this distinction clearly until I had lived on both sides of it, practiced through the consequences of its confusion in thousands of patients, and built an entire medical practice around the imperative to do something about it. Carrera Telehealth and Wellness was not born from a business strategy. It was born from a clinical realization: most people are walking around believing they are fine because no one has ever shown them what "thriving" actually feels like. They have never experienced what their bodies are capable of when given the right conditions. So they accept what they have as the ceiling. It is not.

* * *

For years, I practiced inside systems where the clinical goal was straightforward: rule out emergencies, stabilize presenting symptoms, document the visit, and move on to the next patient. That is what traditional medicine is designed to do. It is not designed to create vitality. It is designed to prevent death. And preventing death is a profoundly important goal — one that medicine achieves with remarkable consistency. But preventing death is not the same as creating a life worth living in a body that fully supports it.

I remember examining patients who were, by every conventional metric, fine. Normal vital signs. Normal laboratory values. Normal imaging. And yet everything about them communicated something different. Their eyes had a particular flatness. Their posture suggested a weight they were carrying that had nothing to do with physical load. Their energy was not just low — it was absent in a way they had stopped noticing, because absence had become their normal. When I asked how they were feeling, the answers were a study in quiet resignation: "I'm managing." "I'm hanging in there." "I guess this is just what getting older feels like."

They were not sick. But they were not well. They were inhabiting the gray zone — what I have come to think of as the medically invisible middle, where dysfunction hides behind normal ranges and symptoms are attributed to stress, age, or lifestyle without further investigation. That zone is where the majority of Americans live. It is where medicine has left them, because medicine, as currently practiced, has no mechanism for finding someone there.

* * *

I was not exempt from this reckoning.

At the height of my career — leading clinical teams, teaching students, speaking nationally, building a practice — I was, by every external measure, succeeding. Internally, I was running on fumes. I was doing what I watched my patients do every day: performing wellness instead of living it. I knew how to function under pressure. I knew how to deliver excellent clinical care even when I was exhausted. What I did not know was how to thrive. And that absence was not a minor gap. For a clinician whose entire professional identity was built around helping others optimize their health, it was a significant clinical and philosophical problem.

That discomfort drove me toward the literature that would ultimately reshape my practice. I began studying longevity medicine and regenerative science with the same systematic attention I applied to clinical pharmacology. Mitochondrial function. Inflammatory pathways. Hormonal regulation across the full lifespan. The mechanisms by which cellular repair occurs — and the conditions under which it fails. I learned that the body does not break down overnight. It whispers for years before it screams. I learned that optimal health is not a genetic lottery. It is a strategy. A learnable, repeatable, measurable strategy.

This became the intellectual and clinical foundation of Carrera Telehealth and Wellness: a practice built not to manage illness, but to build resilience. Not to help patients feel "better," but to help them feel exactly what their bodies are designed to feel when given the right support.

* * *

What Thriving Actually Looks Like

Thriving is not the absence of disease. Thriving is the presence of capacity. The capacity to think clearly under pressure. To recover quickly from physical and emotional stress. To wake in the morning with genuine energy rather than the managed depletion that passes for "okay." To move through daily life with stability, strength, and clarity of purpose. To have a body that supports your goals rather than working against them.

When I evaluate patients, the questions I ask are different from the ones they have grown accustomed to hearing. I am not simply asking whether they have a symptom. I am asking what their lives feel like from the inside. How quickly do you recover after a stressful period? Do you wake rested, or already behind? Do you feel like yourself? Do you have the energy to live the life you long for, versus the reduced version you have learned to accept?

Those questions reveal more about a person's actual health status than any standard laboratory panel. They locate the patient in the spectrum between "not sick" and "thriving" with a precision that a set of normal values cannot.

Optimal health looks like stable energy across the full day. Deep, restorative sleep. Clear cognition and emotional regulation. Strong metabolic flexibility. Low inflammatory burden and rapid recovery from physical demand. Hormonal harmony. Mitochondrial function that produces the energy the body needs. A nervous system that is not chronically locked in sympathetic overdrive.

* * *

Why Most People Never Get There

The primary reason most people never experience what I have just described is not physiological. It is philosophical. They have been conditioned, by years of interaction with a system that treats symptoms rather than systems, to believe that "fine" is the goal. They have been told, explicitly or implicitly, that their fatigue is normal, their brain fog is normal, their weight gain is normal, their disrupted sleep is normal, their declining libido is normal, their anxiety is normal — and that the appropriate response to all of it is acceptance.

Normal, in this framing, means common. And common, in a population where the majority of adults are metabolically compromised, is not a meaningful clinical target.

The wellness industry has compounded the problem with its own category of confusion: an endless cycle of quick fixes, detox protocols, proprietary supplements marketed without clinical evidence, and influencer-driven health advice that sounds authoritative and produces nothing lasting. People are drowning in information. They are starving for wisdom. There is a significant difference between the two.

Wellness is not a product. It is not a trend. It is not something you add to your life for a month and then put away. Wellness is cellular function. Metabolic flexibility. Mitochondrial efficiency. Hormonal alignment. Controlled inflammation. Environmental awareness and deliberate response to environmental exposures. Consistent habits built on a foundation of accurate information about what your specific body needs.

* * *

The Responsibility of Thriving

I built this practice on a principle that the healthcare system rarely articulates clearly: when you thrive, the effects extend beyond yourself. You lead differently. You love differently. You show up differently in every relationship and context that matters to you. The version of yourself that is operating from genuine health and genuine energy is a categorically different presence in the world than the version operating from depletion.

That is not a motivational claim. It is a clinical observation. I have watched it happen in thousands of patients. The transformation in their health produces a transformation in their lives, and the ripple effects extend to everyone around them.

The future of medicine is not symptom management. It is not waiting for a diagnosis. It is not the perpetuation of a model that was built to respond to emergencies and has been asked to do the much harder work of creating health in people who have never been taught what health actually feels like.

The future of medicine is precision, prevention, and optimization. Cellular repair. Metabolic mastery. Nervous system resilience. Personalized, data-driven care that treats the individual rather than the population average.

The future of medicine is thriving. And it begins with the decision to stop settling for anything less.

CHAPTER TEN

The Pillars of Thriving: The Carrera Method™

There comes a moment in most people's lives when they pause long enough to recognize that something fundamental is not working. The exhaustion has crossed a threshold. The weight feels different now — not just physical but accumulated. Sleep has become unreliable. Energy arrives in fragments. The version of themselves they remember — clear-headed, capable, grounded — feels increasingly inaccessible, and they have no precise language for what has changed or why.

If any of that resonates, I want to say this clearly: you are not failing. Your body is not fighting you. It is communicating with you. The problem is not your physiology — the problem is that most people have never been taught how to interpret what their bodies are saying. They have been conditioned to normalize the signals: to accept exhaustion as inevitable, hormonal dysregulation as the price of aging, metabolic dysfunction as a consequence of modern life that cannot be meaningfully addressed without drugs or extraordinary sacrifice.

None of that is true. Your body is designed for balance, strength, clarity, and vitality — at every age and every stage. When you learn to support it correctly, in the right order, with the right tools, everything changes.

This is where The Carrera Method™ begins.

* * *

A Framework Built on Order

The Carrera Method™ is a five-pillar framework for modern integrative wellness. It draws on the evidence base of conventional medicine, the emerging science of longevity and regenerative medicine, and the clinical insights I have gathered across more than two decades of practice in some of the most demanding and diverse healthcare environments in the country.

It is not a quick fix. It is not a detox protocol. It is not a supplement stack or a hormone replacement plan or a fitness program in disguise. It is a sequenced system of interventions, organized around a fundamental clinical truth that most wellness approaches ignore entirely: the body heals in a specific order, and attempting to address any layer of dysfunction without first stabilizing the layers beneath it produces incomplete, unsustainable results.

Most people, when they decide to improve their health, attempt to address everything simultaneously. They overhaul their diet, add a supplement protocol, start a new exercise program, reduce their carbohydrates, increase their protein, buy a sleep tracker, start meditating, and schedule a hormone consultation — all in the same week. The approach is understandable. The biology does not cooperate with it. Attempting to optimize hormones in a body running on cortisol and sympathetic overdrive is like renovating the upper floors of a building with a compromised foundation. The work may be technically sound. It will not hold.

Healing is not about doing more. It is about doing the right things in the right order.

PILLAR 1: Nervous System Regulation — The Foundation of Everything

---

The nervous system is the master regulator of every physiological process in the body. When it is operating in a state of chronic sympathetic activation — the fight-or-flight mode that the modern stress environment produces persistently — every downstream system is compromised. Hormones dysregulate. Inflammatory markers rise. Digestion slows and becomes inefficient. Sleep architecture deteriorates. Cravings for calorie-dense foods intensify as the body attempts to meet a perceived energy emergency. Weight becomes refractory to standard interventions. Mood becomes reactive and difficult to regulate.

None of this is a character deficit. All of it is biology responding predictably to a nervous system that does not feel safe.

The first pillar addresses this directly. Before any other intervention — before nutrition changes, before hormone evaluation, before peptide therapy — the nervous system must be brought into a state in which healing is physiologically possible. This means creating predictable daily rhythms that the body can anchor to. It means prioritizing sleep quality as a non-negotiable clinical priority rather than a lifestyle preference. It means learning to actively shift out of sympathetic dominance through practices that are evidence-based and time-efficient. It means rebuilding the physiological experience of safety in the body.

When the nervous system is regulated, the downstream effects are immediate and measurable. Cortisol patterns normalize. Inflammatory tone decreases. The hormonal environment becomes receptive to optimization rather than resistant to it. Sleep improves in quality and restorative capacity. The body can finally, in the most literal physiological sense, exhale.

PILLAR 2: Metabolic Recalibration — Fueling Strength, Energy, and Longevity

---

Metabolism is the collective term for the biochemical processes by which the body converts nutrients into energy, builds and repairs tissue, and maintains the cellular machinery necessary for life. When these processes are disrupted — by chronic stress, by dietary patterns that destabilize blood glucose, by insufficient protein intake, by sedentary behavior, by environmental toxin exposure — the downstream effects are pervasive: unstable energy, altered body composition, intensified cravings, disrupted mood, and accelerated biological aging.

Metabolic recalibration does not mean restriction. It means support. Protein-forward nutrition that preserves and builds lean muscle mass. Dietary patterns that promote glucose stability and reduce the insulin spikes that drive fat storage and inflammatory activation. Adequate hydration with appropriate electrolyte balance. Mitochondrial support through targeted micronutrient repletion. Strategic reduction of the inflammatory dietary inputs that are ubiquitous in the standard American food environment.

This is where most patients begin to feel the first tangible shift. Energy stabilizes. Mood improves before hormones are ever addressed. Body composition begins to respond. Cravings diminish as blood sugar regulation normalizes. The patient who said "I finally feel like myself again" after two weeks of metabolic support is reporting a real, measurable physiological change — not a placebo effect.

PILLAR 3: Hormonal Harmony — Restoring the Body's Natural Rhythm

---

Hormones are regulatory molecules that coordinate virtually every biological function: metabolism, reproduction, mood, cognition, sleep, immune response, cardiovascular function, bone density, and cellular repair. Hormonal imbalance is not a condition limited to perimenopause or andropause — it is a spectrum of dysfunction that can develop at any age, in any body, in response to chronic stress, nutritional deficiency, environmental exposures, or the natural transitions of the lifespan.

For women, the relevant hormonal landscape often involves estrogen, progesterone, thyroid function, DHEA, and cortisol — with particular complexity during the perimenopause and menopause transitions, which represent not simply the cessation of reproductive function but a full-system endocrine recalibration with wide-ranging effects on metabolic, cardiovascular, cognitive, and psychological health. For men, the parallel conversation centers on testosterone, DHEA, cortisol, thyroid, and insulin sensitivity — with testosterone decline beginning as early as the third decade and accelerating substantially under conditions of chronic stress, poor sleep, and metabolic dysfunction.

Hormonal evaluation and optimization is the third pillar — not the first. This sequencing is not arbitrary. Attempting to balance hormones in a body that is running on cortisol and metabolically compromised is like trying to calibrate a precision instrument on a table that is vibrating. The instrument cannot be accurately set until the environment is stable. Hormones work best when the nervous system and metabolic foundation are already supporting them.

When the first two pillars are in place and hormonal assessment reveals deficiencies or imbalances, targeted optimization can produce results that are genuinely transformative: restored energy, improved cognitive clarity, recovered libido, stabilized mood, enhanced body composition, and a measurable reduction in the inflammatory and metabolic markers that predict long-term disease risk.

PILLAR 4: Inflammation Reduction and Cellular Repair

Inflammation is the body's primary defense and repair mechanism. Acute inflammation — the kind that responds to infection or injury and resolves when the threat has passed — is essential and adaptive. Chronic low-grade inflammation, the kind that persists in the absence of an acute threat, is among the most significant drivers of premature aging and chronic disease that we know of. It is implicated in cardiovascular disease, type 2 diabetes, neurodegenerative conditions, autoimmune disorders, and malignancy. And it is staggeringly common in the modern population.

The drivers of chronic inflammation are multiple and often cumulative: a diet dominated by processed foods and refined carbohydrates, persistent psychological stress, disrupted sleep, sedentary behavior, dysbiotic gut microbiome, environmental toxin exposure, and chronic infections that have been inadequately addressed. Identifying and systematically addressing these inputs is the clinical work of the fourth pillar.

Gut health occupies a central position in this work. The intestinal microbiome is not simply a digestive organ — it is a critical mediator of immune function, neurotransmitter production, metabolic regulation, and systemic inflammatory tone. When the gut ecosystem is disrupted, the consequences are distributed throughout every system in the body. Restoring gut integrity through targeted nutritional and supplemental intervention creates conditions in which systemic inflammation can meaningfully decrease.

Alongside gut repair, the fourth pillar addresses micronutrient repletion, mitochondrial support, and strategic reduction of the environmental and dietary inputs that sustain inflammatory activation. When this work is done well, patients describe a quality of change that is qualitatively different from the energy improvements they experienced in pillar two: a decrease in baseline pain and stiffness, accelerated recovery from physical exertion, improved skin quality and appearance, enhanced cognitive clarity, and a general sense of biological ease that they had either never experienced or had not felt in years.

PILLAR 5: Personalized Optimization — Advanced Tools for Advanced Goals

The fifth pillar is where the tools that have received the most popular attention — peptides, regenerative therapies, advanced hormone optimization, genetic insights, longevity protocols — are applied. This sequencing is deliberate and clinically essential. These are powerful tools. They are also tools that work by supporting and amplifying what the body is already doing — which means they require a body that is already functioning at a foundational level of health to produce the results they can produce. Applied to an unprepared system, they become expensive symptomatic interventions at best. At worst, they can add complexity to dysfunction that has not been addressed at its root.

When the first four pillars are in place, personalized optimization can achieve outcomes that genuinely approach what the word "optimal" means: hormonal levels calibrated to the individual's biology and life stage, not simply to population reference ranges. Peptide therapies that support specific regenerative, metabolic, or neurological goals. Targeted supplementation informed by genetic and laboratory data rather than general recommendations. Longevity-oriented monitoring that tracks biological age markers over time and adjusts the protocol in response to what the data shows. Telehealth-guided care that provides access to this level of clinical sophistication without the barriers of geography or institutional gatekeeping.

This is what personalized medicine means — not personalized in the marketing sense but personalized in the clinical sense: built around the specific biology, history, goals, and circumstances of a single individual.

The Order That Works

The sequence of The Carrera Method™ is not a stylistic preference. It reflects how the body heals. Stabilize the nervous system. Correct metabolic foundations. Balance hormones. Reduce inflammation and repair cellular function. Then, and only then, apply advanced optimization tools with the full confidence that the system beneath them is prepared to use them.

The most common mistake I see in patients who have attempted to improve their health without guidance is skipping the early pillars and beginning with the last one. They invest in peptides or hormone therapy or expensive supplement protocols before their nervous system is regulated, their metabolism is supported, or their inflammatory burden has been meaningfully addressed. The interventions may be clinically sound. The results will be partial, because the foundation required to translate them into lasting change is not yet in place.

The Heart of the Method

At its center, The Carrera Method™ is not about any specific intervention or protocol. It is about a relationship — between the patient and their own body. My job is not to heal you. My job is to give you the information, the tools, and the clinical support to understand what your body is communicating, to address the conditions that are preventing it from functioning optimally, and to build the physiological foundation on which genuine, sustained vitality becomes possible.

Your body is not broken. It is not your enemy. Every symptom is information. Every imbalance points toward something that can be identified, addressed, and resolved. The path from where you are to where you are capable of being is not mysterious — it is systematic. It requires clarity about where to start, commitment to working through the layers in the right order, and support from someone with the clinical knowledge to guide you through it.

This is your moment — woman or man — to reclaim your health from the inside out. Your body is ready. Your future is waiting. And The Carrera Method™ is here to guide you home.

CHAPTER ELEVEN

EPINUTRITION: HOW FOOD REWRITES YOUR GENES

Food is not just fuel.

Food is biological information.

Every meal you eat delivers molecular instructions that interact with your cells, your enzymes, your microbiome, and — most importantly — your epigenome, the dynamic layer of biochemical switches that determines how your genes behave.

This is the foundation of epigenetics and epinutrition: the science of how nutrients, bioactive compounds, and environmental inputs regulate gene expression without altering your DNA sequence.

Your DNA is the hardware.

Your environment — especially your nutrition — is the software.

And the software is far more powerful than most people realize.

Epigenetics explains why two people with the same genes can have completely different health outcomes. It explains why identical twins age differently, why some people thrive under stress while others break down, and why lifestyle can override genetic risk in profound ways.

It also explains one of the most fascinating biological phenomena in nature: how a queen bee and a worker bee can share the same DNA yet become entirely different creatures.

* * *

THE QUEEN BEE VS. WORKER BEE: THE ULTIMATE EPIGENETIC STORY

In the beehive, the queen bee and the worker bees are genetically identical.

Same genome. Same blueprint. Same potential.

Yet their lives diverge dramatically:

- The queen is larger, fertile, lives 10–20 times longer, and has a completely different physiology and role.
- Worker bees are smaller, sterile, shorter-lived, and biologically programmed for labor.

So what creates this dramatic difference?

Nutrition.

The queen bee is fed royal jelly, a nutrient-dense secretion rich in proteins, lipids, and bioactive compounds that act like epigenetic "instructions." Royal jelly does not change her DNA — it changes how her DNA is expressed. It activates queen-specific genes and silences worker-specific ones.

This single nutritional input determines: her size, her fertility, her longevity, her hormonal profile, her metabolic rate, and her entire biological destiny.

Same genetic hardware.

Different nutritional software.

Completely different outcome.

This is epigenetics in its purest form.

* * *

THE 30/70 RULE: GENES ARE THE PIANO, LIFESTYLE IS THE PIANIST

In humans, the same principle applies.

Approximately 30 percent of your genetic expression is fixed — the part you inherit and cannot change. But the remaining 70 percent is influenced by environment, including:

- Nutrition
- Stress
- Sleep
- Movement
- Toxins
- Microbiome

- Light exposure
- Hormones
- Emotional environment
- Social connection

This means your daily choices are constantly shaping your biological future. You are not a passive passenger in your genetics. You are an active participant.

And food is one of the most powerful levers you have.

* * *

EPINUTRITION: THE NUTRITIONAL LANGUAGE OF YOUR GENES

Epinutrition is the study of how nutrients and bioactive compounds influence gene expression. It focuses on two major categories of nutritional signals:

- Methyl Donors — the biochemical "switches"

- Epibiotics — the signaling molecules that guide gene behavior

Together, they form the nutritional language your body uses to regulate genetic expression.

* * *

METHYL DONORS: THE BIOCHEMICAL SWITCHES OF GENE EXPRESSION

Methyl donors are nutrients that provide methyl groups — tiny chemical tags (CH_3) that attach to DNA and influence whether genes are turned on or off. This process is called DNA methylation, and it is one of the most important epigenetic mechanisms in the human body.

Why Methylation Matters

Methylation influences:

- Detoxification
- Hormone metabolism
- Neurotransmitter production

- Inflammation
- Mitochondrial function
- Cellular repair
- Immune regulation
- Mood and cognition
- Cardiovascular health
- Aging

When methylation is optimal, your system runs smoothly. When it is impaired, everything from mood to metabolism can suffer.

Key Methyl Donors

The major nutritional methyl donors include:

- Methionine
- Folate (B9)
- Vitamin B12

- Choline
- Betaine (TMG)
- Vitamin B6 (supports methylation pathways)

These nutrients provide the raw materials your body needs to maintain healthy gene regulation.

What Happens When You Don't Get Enough?

Low methyl donor intake can lead to:

- Poor detoxification
- Elevated homocysteine
- Fatigue
- Mood instability
- Hormonal imbalance
- Impaired liver function
- Cognitive decline

- Accelerated aging
- Increased inflammation

In other words: without methyl donors, your epigenetic system lacks the resources to do its job.

Food Sources of Methyl Donors

- Eggs
- Salmon and sardines
- Leafy greens
- Liver
- Beets
- Legumes
- Nuts and seeds
- Avocado

These foods do not just nourish your body — they help regulate your genetic expression.

* * *

EPIBIOTICS: THE SIGNALING MOLECULES THAT GUIDE GENE BEHAVIOR

If methyl donors are the "switches," epibiotics are the signals. Epibiotics are compounds — mostly from plants and fermented foods — that act as epigenetic messengers. They do not provide methyl groups; instead, they influence the enzymes and pathways that determine how genes behave.

Major Categories of Epibiotics

Polyphenols

Found in berries, green tea, cacao, olives, herbs, spices, and deeply colored plants. Polyphenols can reduce inflammation, improve mitochondrial function, support detoxification, enhance metabolic flexibility, and protect DNA from oxidative stress. They are some of the most powerful epigenetic modulators in nature.

Omega-3 Fatty Acids

EPA and DHA influence gene expression related to inflammation, brain function, cardiovascular health, and cell membrane fluidity. They help shift the body toward an anti-inflammatory state.

Fermented Foods and Postbiotics

Your microbiome produces epigenetically active compounds such as short-chain fatty acids (SCFAs), butyrate, propionate, and lactate. These compounds directly influence gene expression in the gut and beyond.

Sulforaphane and Cruciferous Compounds

Found in broccoli sprouts, kale, cabbage, and Brussels sprouts. They activate detoxification genes and support cellular resilience.

How Epibiotics Work

Epibiotics influence histone acetylation, DNA methylation patterns, inflammatory gene expression, antioxidant pathways, mitochondrial biogenesis, and cellular repair mechanisms. They are like the "coaches" of your genome — guiding, directing, and optimizing performance.

* * *

THE SYNERGY: HOW METHYL DONORS + EPIBIOTICS WORK TOGETHER

Methyl donors provide the biochemical hardware. Epibiotics provide the software instructions. Together, they create a powerful synergy that supports:

- Healthy aging
- Better metabolic function
- Improved cognitive performance
- Lower inflammation
- Enhanced detoxification
- Stronger mitochondrial health
- Greater resilience to stress
- More stable mood and energy

This is not theoretical. This is measurable biology.

* * *

EPINUTRITION AND LONGEVITY: TURNING ON THE GENES THAT KEEP YOU YOUNG

Longevity is not just about adding years to your life — it is about adding life to your years. Epinutrition influences longevity through several key pathways:

1. Sirtuins

These are longevity genes that regulate DNA repair, mitochondrial function, inflammation, and metabolic efficiency. Epibiotics like resveratrol, quercetin, and fisetin activate sirtuins.

2. AMPK Activation

AMPK is the metabolic "master switch" that enhances fat burning, cellular repair, and mitochondrial biogenesis. Compounds like berberine, green tea catechins, and fasting activate AMPK.

3. mTOR Modulation

mTOR regulates growth and aging. Balanced mTOR activity supports longevity. Nutrients like polyphenols and omega-3s help modulate mTOR.

4. Detoxification Pathways

Sulforaphane and cruciferous compounds activate Nrf2, the body's detoxification and antioxidant master regulator.

5. Inflammation Control

Epibiotics help silence inflammatory genes and activate anti-inflammatory pathways.

* * *

EPINUTRITION AND METABOLIC HEALTH

Your metabolism is not just about calories — it is about cellular communication. Epinutrition improves metabolic health by:

- Enhancing insulin sensitivity
- Reducing chronic inflammation
- Supporting mitochondrial function

- Improving lipid metabolism
- Regulating appetite hormones
- Supporting liver detoxification

This is why two people can eat the same diet and have completely different metabolic outcomes. Their epigenetic environment determines how their body responds.

* * *

EPINUTRITION AND MENTAL HEALTH

Your brain is one of the most epigenetically sensitive organs in the body. Methyl donors support neurotransmitter production, myelin formation, cognitive clarity, and mood stability. Epibiotics support neuroplasticity, neuroprotection, reduced neuroinflammation, and improved stress resilience.

This is why nutrition is one of the most powerful tools for mental well-being.

* * *

EPINUTRITION AND HORMONE BALANCE

Hormones are deeply influenced by epigenetic signals. Methyl donors help metabolize estrogen, cortisol, adrenal hormones, and thyroid hormones. Epibiotics help regulate inflammatory pathways, insulin signaling, and receptor sensitivity. Together, they create a hormonal environment that supports vitality, energy, and balance.

* * *

THE TAKEAWAY: YOU ARE THE ARCHITECT OF YOUR BIOLOGY

You cannot change the DNA you were born with. But you can absolutely change how that DNA is expressed.

Food is one of the most powerful tools you have. Just like the queen bee, your biology is shaped not only by your genes but by the signals you feed them.

Epinutrition is the science — and the opportunity — to influence your genetic destiny through intentional nourishment.

You are not at the mercy of your genes. You are the architect of your biology.

* * *

CLINICAL CASE STUDY: REWRITING BIOLOGY THROUGH EPINUTRITION

Patient: "Maria," 47-year-old female

Presenting Concerns: Fatigue, weight gain, brain fog, elevated inflammatory markers, and a strong family history of metabolic disease.

Maria came into the clinic frustrated. She exercised regularly, ate what she believed was a "healthy diet," and yet she felt like her body was working against her. Her mother had developed Type 2 diabetes in her early fifties, and Maria feared she was headed down the same path.

Her labs revealed:

- Elevated homocysteine
- Low-normal B12

- Suboptimal folate
- High-sensitivity CRP mildly elevated
- Early signs of insulin resistance
- Low omega-3 index
- Low dietary polyphenol intake based on nutrition recall

Nothing was catastrophic. But everything pointed toward a body under epigenetic stress.

Maria's story is common: she was not dealing with a single disease. She was dealing with dysregulated gene expression driven by years of low-grade inflammation, nutrient insufficiency, and environmental stressors. This is where epinutrition becomes powerful.

* * *

Understanding Maria Through an Epigenetic Lens

Maria's genetics were not her destiny. They were her blueprint. But her environment — her nutrition, stress, sleep, and lifestyle — was shaping how that blueprint was being read.

Her elevated homocysteine suggested impaired methylation. Her low omega-3 index suggested inflammatory gene pathways were overactive. Her low polyphenol intake meant she lacked the epibiotic signals that help regulate detoxification, mitochondrial function, and cellular repair.

In other words, her epigenetic "software" needed an upgrade. Just like the queen bee and worker bee, Maria's biology was responding to the signals she was feeding it.

The Epinutritional Approach

The goal was not to "treat" a disease. The goal was to optimize her epigenetic environment so her genes could express themselves in a healthier way. Her plan focused on the two major food groups of epinutrition:

1. Methyl Donors (the biochemical switches)

These nutrients support DNA methylation, detoxification, neurotransmitter balance, and hormone metabolism. Maria's nutrition recall showed low intake of folate-rich leafy greens, choline-rich foods like eggs, B12-rich proteins, and betaine-rich foods like beets. Her body simply did not have the raw materials needed for optimal gene regulation.

2. Epibiotics (the signaling molecules)

These compounds help guide gene expression toward anti-inflammatory, antioxidant, and longevity pathways. Maria's diet was low in polyphenols, omega-3 fatty acids, cruciferous vegetables, and fermented foods. Her genes were not receiving the signals they needed to activate protective pathways.

The Shift: Rewriting Her Biological Story

Over the next several months, Maria focused on increasing methyl donor-rich foods, adding omega-3-rich seafood, incorporating deeply colored fruits and vegetables, adding cruciferous vegetables for sulforaphane, including fermented foods for microbiome-driven epigenetic signals, and supporting sleep, stress reduction, and movement.

These were not extreme interventions. They were targeted epigenetic inputs.

What Happened Next

Within 8 to 12 weeks, Maria reported improved energy, clearer thinking, more stable mood, better metabolic flexibility, reduced cravings, and improved exercise recovery. Her follow-up labs showed homocysteine trending down, improved B12 and folate status, lower inflammatory markers, and an improved omega-3 index.

Nothing about her DNA had changed. But her gene expression had. Her biology began behaving differently because her environment was different.

* * *

The Queen Bee Analogy in Human Form

Maria's case mirrors the queen bee phenomenon: same DNA, different nutritional signals, different biological outcome. Her "worker bee" physiology — fatigue, inflammation, metabolic strain — was not a fixed destiny. It reflected the signals her body had been receiving.

Once those signals changed, her biology changed. This is the power of epinutrition.

* * *

Why This Case Matters

Maria's story is not unique. It is the story of millions of people who feel like their body is working against them, when, their epigenome is simply responding to the inputs it receives.

Epinutrition reframes the conversation: from "What disease do you have?" to "What signals are your genes receiving?" It shifts the focus from genetics to gene behavior, from inevitability to empowerment.

Maria did not need a new genome. She needed a new environment. And when she changed the inputs, her biology responded.

* * *

The Takeaway

This case illustrates the central truth of epinutrition: your genes are not your destiny. Your daily choices are.

Just like the queen bee, your biology is shaped not only by your DNA but by the signals you feed it. Methyl donors provide the switches. Epibiotics provide the instructions. Your lifestyle provides the context. Together, they determine how your genes express themselves — and ultimately, how you feel, function, and age.

CHAPTER TWELVE

THE F-A-C-E-I-T PROTOCOL: YOUR BLUEPRINT FOR LONGEVITY, PERFORMANCE & EPIGENETIC HEALTH

You are not meant to simply age — you are meant to evolve.

The F-A-C-E-I-T Protocol is your roadmap for doing exactly that.

Originally developed by orthopedic surgeon Dr. Vonda Wright, the F-A-C-E framework reframed aging as an active, trainable process. Expanded here into a six-pillar system that integrates biomechanics, movement science, epigenetics, and regenerative therapeutics, it represents a complete blueprint for human performance, metabolic health, and cellular longevity.

Here is what it stands for:

- F — Flexibility
- A — Activity
- C — Carry a Load
- E — Equilibrium
- I — Intracellular Activation (Epinutrition)
- T — Therapeutic Biologics (Peptides, Stem Cells, Exosomes, PRP)

Each pillar builds on the others. Together, they help you rewrite your biology — from the way you move to the way your genes express themselves.

THE PHILOSOPHY OF F-A-C-E-I-T

Your body is not a fixed structure — it is a dynamic, adaptive system. Every day, your cells are listening to the signals you send them: how you move, how you nourish yourself, how you recover, how you think, how you sleep, how you manage stress, and how you fuel your epigenome.

These signals determine whether your biology moves toward resilience or degeneration. The F-A-C-E-I-T protocol helps you send the right ones — the ones that support longevity, mobility, metabolic health, and cellular repair.

* * *

F — FLEXIBILITY: RESTORING MOVEMENT FREEDOM

Flexibility is the foundation of youthful movement. Without it, strength becomes limited, balance becomes compromised, and activity becomes painful. Think of flexibility as your body's language of freedom — the ability to move with ease, grace, and confidence.

Why Flexibility Declines

As you age, collagen cross-linking increases, fascia stiffens, and joints lose their natural range of motion. Sedentary habits, inflammation, and repetitive stress accelerate this process. But you can reverse it.

Your Flexibility System

1. Stretching Exercises

Make stretching part of your daily rhythm. Use dynamic stretches before activity, static stretches afterward, and deeper contract-relax (PNF) stretches for mobility. Even five minutes a day keeps your joints supple, and your fascia hydrated.

2. Yoga

Yoga blends flexibility, breathwork, balance, and mindfulness. It restores fascial elasticity, strengthens your core, and calms your nervous system. If you are under stress or feel tight and tense, yoga is medicine.

3. Pilates

Pilates strengthens the deep stabilizing muscles that support mobility. It improves posture, spinal alignment, and controlled movement. If you sit often or struggle with back tension, Pilates helps you rebuild your foundation.

Flexibility is not optional — it is your gateway to movement freedom.

* * *

A — ACTIVITY: MOTION IS MEDICINE

You were designed to move. Movement is not a chore — it is a biological requirement.

Your Activity Prescription

Commit to at least 30 minutes of activity, three times a week. Choose what you enjoy — brisk walking, cycling, swimming, rowing, dancing — anything that elevates your heart rate and makes you feel alive.

Cardiac Acceleration: Challenge Your Heart

To truly condition your cardiovascular system, add short bursts of intensity. Here is your formula:

- 30-second sprint intervals
- 3 times during each workout
- 3 days per week

You can sprint, row, cycle, swim, or climb stairs — whatever fits your body. These brief accelerations challenge your heart, lungs, and mitochondria, improving VO_2 max, insulin sensitivity, and metabolic flexibility. It is not punishment — it is precision training for longevity.

* * *

C — CARRY A LOAD: BUILDING THE MUSCLE THAT PROTECTS YOUR FUTURE

Muscle is your metabolic currency. It is what keeps you strong, stable, and independent. You do not need a gym to build it — start with what you have: your body weight, five-pound dumbbells, or even water bottles.

Start Where You Are

Consistency matters more than perfection. Begin small, then progress weekly — even one pound at a time.

Your Foundational Strength Moves

Push-Ups

Start with wall or countertop push-ups and progress to full ones. They build your chest, shoulders, triceps, and core.

Squats

Begin with chair squats, then add dumbbells. Squats strengthen your glutes, quads, and hamstrings — the muscles that keep you mobile.

Lunges

Start with static lunges, then add weight. They build balance, hip stability, and functional strength.

Calf Raises

Progress from two-foot to single-leg raises, then add weight. Strong calves improve gait and reduce fall risk.

Hanging From a Bar

Grip strength predicts longevity. Hang for five to ten seconds, then add time or a backpack for resistance. It strengthens your shoulders, back, and core while decompressing your spine.

The Suitcase Drill

Think about lifting your carry-on overhead on a plane. Start with an empty suitcase, practice the motion, then gradually add items. This trains real-world strength — the kind that keeps you capable and confident.

Progressive Overload

Add a little more each week — one pound, one rep, one second. Small increases compound into major strength gains.

* * *

E — EQUILIBRIUM: TRAINING YOUR BRAIN-BODY CONNECTION

Balance is a skill — and it is trainable. It is one of the first abilities to decline with age, but one of the easiest to restore. Poor equilibrium increases fall risk and limits confidence. Training it strengthens your nervous system, coordination, and reaction time.

Your Daily Balance Practice

Stand on One Foot While Brushing Your Teeth

Hold the counter lightly at first, then progress to no hands. This simple habit trains your stabilizers and proprioception.

Jump Rope

Start with ten to twenty seconds. It improves rhythm, coordination, and cardiovascular health.

Hop on One Foot

Do five to ten small hops on a soft surface. It builds tendon elasticity and ankle stability.

Close Your Eyes (Advanced)

Once you are steady, try balancing with eyes closed. It forces your brain to rely on proprioception and the inner ear. Always practice in a safe environment and work up gradually.

Balance is your neurological glue — it holds everything together.

* * *

I — INTRACELLULAR ACTIVATION: TURNING YOUR GENES ON AND OFF

This is where the protocol becomes revolutionary. The "I" stands for Intracellular Activation — influencing gene expression through epinutrition.

Movement changes your body from the outside in. Nutrition changes it from the inside out.

Methyl Donors: The Biochemical Switches

These nutrients provide methyl groups that regulate DNA methylation — turning genes on or off. Include foods rich in folate, B12, choline, methionine, betaine, and B6. They support detoxification, neurotransmitter balance, hormone metabolism, and cellular repair.

Epibiotics: The Signaling Molecules

Epibiotics guide gene expression toward anti-inflammatory and longevity pathways. Include polyphenols (berries, green tea, cacao), omega-3 fatty acids, fermented foods, cruciferous vegetables, and plant bioactives.

Together, methyl donors and epibiotics create an intracellular environment that supports healthy aging, improved metabolism, and stronger immunity. You are not just feeding your body — you are programming your genes.

* * *

T — THERAPEUTIC BIOLOGICS: AMPLIFYING YOUR BODY'S REPAIR SYSTEM

The final pillar represents Therapeutic Biologics — advanced regenerative tools that support tissue repair, cellular communication, and optimal performance. These therapies do not replace lifestyle; they amplify it.

Peptide Therapy

Supports tissue repair, inflammation control, mitochondrial function, and recovery.

Stem Cells

Offer regenerative potential and anti-inflammatory effects for joint and tissue health.

Exosomes

Enhance cellular communication and healing through growth factors and signaling molecules.

PRP (Platelet-Rich Plasma)

Delivers concentrated growth factors for tendon, ligament, and skin rejuvenation.

These are accelerators — helping your body do what it is already designed to do: heal.

* * *

THE SYNERGY: HOW ALL SIX PILLARS WORK TOGETHER

The F-A-C-E-I-T protocol is not six separate strategies — it is one integrated system.

- Flexibility improves mobility.
- Activity improves metabolism.
- Carrying a load builds strength and bone density.
- Equilibrium enhances neurological stability.

- Intracellular activation optimizes gene expression.
- Therapeutic biologics accelerate repair and regeneration.

Together, they create a 360-degree model of human performance and longevity. This is not about "anti-aging." This is about pro-function, pro-vitality, and pro-resilience.

* * *

CONCLUSION

YOUR BODY IS NOT THE PROBLEM – IT'S THE MESSENGER

Your body is not broken. It is communicating.

Every symptom is a signal. Every imbalance is a message. Every struggle is an invitation to understand yourself more deeply.

The Carrera Method™ gives you the roadmap. You bring the willingness. Together, they create the transformation.

This is your moment — woman or man — to reclaim your health from the inside out. To step into a life where you feel strong, clear, energized, and aligned.

Your body is ready. Your future is waiting.

And The Carrera Method™ is here to guide you home.

CHAPTER THIRTEEN

THE FUTURE OF MEDICINE

If the last decade has taught us anything, it is that medicine is changing faster than most people realize. The old model — the one built on rushed appointments, symptom-based treatment, and one-size-fits-all protocols — is quietly collapsing. Patients feel it. Providers feel it. The entire system feels it. People are tired of being told their labs are "normal" when they feel anything but normal. They are tired of being dismissed, rushed, or given a prescription instead of an explanation. They are tired of feeling like their health is something that happens to them instead of something they can actively shape. And they are right to want more.

The future of medicine is not about more pills, more procedures, or more complexity. It is about precision, personalization, prevention, and partnership. It is about giving people the tools, insights, and support they need to understand their bodies — and to thrive in them.

* * *

The Next Decade: A New Era of Medicine

We are standing at the edge of a transformation that will redefine how women and men experience healthcare. Over the next decade, medicine will shift from reactive to proactive, from generalized to personalized, from symptom-focused to system-focused, from episodic care to continuous care, and from provider-centered to patient-empowered. Let's look at what each of those shifts means.

For most of modern history, healthcare has operated on a simple formula: wait until something goes wrong, treat the problem, hope it does not return. This model is outdated, expensive, and ineffective. The future flips the script. Instead of waiting for disease, we will identify risk patterns early, track biomarkers over time, use genetics and epigenetics to predict vulnerabilities, and address inflammation before it becomes disease. Continuous glucose monitors, wearable devices, epigenetic hair analysis, microbiome mapping, and advanced hormone panels are already giving us real-time insight into how the body is functioning. In the next ten years, these tools will become standard.

The era of "take this, it works for most people" is ending. Modern science has established that two people can eat the same meal and have completely different glucose responses, take the same medication and have opposite reactions, follow the same diet and see entirely different results. Personalized medicine uses genetics, epigenetics, hormone mapping, microbiome analysis, metabolic data, lifestyle patterns, and environmental exposures to create protocols as unique as the person they are designed for. This is where peptides, hormone optimization, and precision supplementation shine — not as shortcuts, but as targeted tools.

Symptoms are not the problem. They are the signal. The future of medicine will focus on the systems that drive health: the nervous system, the endocrine system, the metabolic system, the immune system, the gut-brain axis, the mitochondrial network. Instead of asking how we suppress this symptom, we will ask what system is signaling distress, and why. This is the foundation of The Carrera Method™, and it is the direction medicine is moving globally.

Telehealth is not a trend. It is the future. In the next ten years, most routine care will be virtual, monitoring will be wearable and automated, providers will track trends instead of snapshots, and patients will have access to their data in real time. Communication will be ongoing instead of appointment-based. Patients will no longer wait months for answers. They will have support when they need it.

* * *

The Rise of Peptides: Why They Matter

Peptides are short chains of amino acids — essentially small fragments of proteins — that act as signaling molecules in the body. They tell cells what to do, how to repair, when to recover, and how to function more efficiently. Your body already makes hundreds of peptides naturally, and they regulate healing, inflammation, metabolism, hormones, immune function, brain chemistry, energy production, and tissue repair. Peptide therapy uses synthetic versions of naturally occurring peptides to support or enhance these processes.

In the next ten years, peptides will become one of the most important tools in modern medicine because they work with the body's natural signaling, have targeted and predictable effects, support cellular repair, improve metabolic function, enhance recovery, reduce inflammation, and support cognitive health. Peptides are not magic. They are biology, refined. And as research expands, they will play major roles in longevity medicine, regenerative therapies, metabolic optimization, hormone support, injury recovery, immune modulation, and cognitive enhancement.

A Critical Word on Peptide Safety

Not all peptides are created equal, and the regulatory landscape matters enormously. You will encounter the term RUO — Research Use Only — throughout discussions of peptide therapy. RUO means the peptide is not FDA-approved for human use, is not approved as a drug, supplement, or treatment, and is intended for laboratory research only. It must be handled by licensed medical professionals and must not be purchased, injected, or used by the general public without proper medical oversight.

This is not a technicality. It is a legal and safety boundary. Many peptides circulating online — especially on social media — are unregulated, impure, incorrectly labeled, incorrectly stored, incorrectly reconstituted, incorrectly dosed, or contaminated. This is why RUO peptides must only be used under the supervision of a licensed medical provider who understands pharmacology, physiology, contraindications, side-effect profiles, drug interactions, lab monitoring, and clinical red flags.

We are living in a time when social media influencers are giving advice on peptides, hormones, injections, and so-called biohacking protocols. Most of these individuals are not licensed medical providers. They have no training in physiology, no understanding of pharmacology, and no concept of contraindications or long-term risks. And yet they speak with confidence. The real-world consequences of following influencer protocols include anxiety, palpitations, tachycardia, insomnia, panic attacks, hormonal disruption, blood sugar instability, and emergency room visits. Not because peptides are inherently dangerous, but because misuse is dangerous. Peptides are not toys. They are not wellness fads. They are biological signals that can profoundly affect your body, and they belong in the hands of licensed medical providers, not content creators.

* * *

What Patients Should Demand from Their Providers

The future of medicine is not just about what providers offer. It is about what patients insist on. You deserve a provider who listens, who asks questions, and who sees you as a whole person. You should understand your labs, your options, and your plan — not feel confused or dismissed. Your care should reflect your biology, not a generic template. You deserve a provider who looks deeper than symptoms, who collaborates with you as a partner rather than an authority figure, who gives you access to modern tools and precision medicine, and who respects your lived experience. Your symptoms matter. Your intuition matters. Patients are no longer passive recipients of care. They are active participants, and the future of medicine will honor that.

The future belongs to those who are willing to evolve — both the providers who embrace innovation and the patients who refuse to settle.

CHAPTER FOURTEEN

YOUR DNA IS NOT YOUR DESTINY - YOUR DAILY DECISIONS ARE

There is a myth that has held people hostage for decades: the belief that your genetics determine your future. That your family history is your fate. That if your mother had diabetes, you will too. If your father had heart disease, it is inevitable. If your grandmother struggled with weight, it is in your genes and there is nothing to be done about it. Modern science — specifically the field of epigenetics — has shattered that myth.

Your DNA is the piano. Your lifestyle is the pianist. Two people can have the same instrument, the music produced depends on how it is played. You are not a prisoner of your genetics. You are the architect of your biology. Your DNA is the blueprint. Your habits are the builders. Your environment is the architect. Your choices are the contractors. Your biometrics are the feedback system. And the truth is simple: you cannot change your DNA, but you can absolutely change how your DNA behaves. This is where measurement becomes power.

* * *

Epigenetics: Queen Bee vs Worker Bee

Epigenetics is the study of how your environment, lifestyle, stress, sleep, nutrition, and habits influence the expression of your genes. Think of your genes as a piano. Epigenetics is the pianist. You may have inherited the instrument, but you decide the music. Epigenetic research shows that stress can turn genes on, sleep can turn genes off, inflammation can activate disease pathways, movement can silence harmful patterns, nutrition can repair cellular signaling, trauma can alter gene expression, and healing practices can reverse those changes. Your DNA is not a sentence. It is a set of possibilities.

Your daily habits determine which possibilities become reality.

One of the most compelling illustrations of epigenetics in nature is the honeybee. Queen bees and worker bees have identical DNA, yet they become completely different organisms. The queen grows larger, lives years longer, becomes fertile, and can lay up to two thousand eggs a day. Worker bees stay smaller, are mostly sterile, and live only a few weeks. The difference? Nutrition. Future queen bees are fed royal jelly, which acts as an epigenetic signal that changes gene expression. Same genetics. Radically different biological outcome. While human epigenetics is more complex, the principle stands: what you feed your body — in food, in rest, in stress, in movement — influences which genes are expressed and how.

Epinutrition: Food as a Signal

The emerging field of epinutrition explores how dietary compounds influence gene expression. Two categories of nutrients are central to this work. Methyl donors — found in eggs, meat, leafy greens, liver, and beets — are the ink in the pen that writes the expression for your genes. They help regulate DNA function and methylation pathways. Epibiotics — found in colorful plants, berries, broccoli, coffee, dark chocolate, fermented foods, and omega-3-rich fish — act as signals that influence inflammation, cellular repair, and gene expression. Your genes may be the blueprint, but your nutrition helps determine how that blueprint is read. You cannot completely change your DNA, but your daily choices influence how your body expresses it. That is a profound form of agency.

* * *

Why Biometrics Matter: Data Is the New Medicine

You cannot improve what you cannot see. You cannot change what you do not track. You cannot master what you do not measure. Biometrics are not simply numbers — they are your body speaking in data. They tell you how you are aging, how you are recovering, how you are adapting, how you are inflamed, how you are sleeping, how you are metabolizing, and how your nervous system is coping. Without biometrics, you are guessing. With biometrics, you are leading.

Labs are not about diagnosing disease. They are about understanding patterns. When used correctly, they reveal inflammation markers, hormonal rhythms, thyroid efficiency, metabolic flexibility, blood sugar stability, liver detox capacity, immune balance, nutrient status, and cardiovascular risk. You would never drive a car without a dashboard. You should never navigate your health without one either.

Two laboratory markers deserve particular attention because they are foundational and often overlooked. Homocysteine is an amino acid involved in methylation — a process that affects detoxification, DNA repair, hormone metabolism, neurotransmitter production, inflammation control, and cardiovascular health. When elevated, it can signal B-vitamin insufficiency, increased inflammation, impaired detox pathways, and higher cardiovascular strain. It does not diagnose disease, but it reveals stress on your system long before symptoms appear. ApoB, or Apolipoprotein B, is considered by many cardiometabolic experts to be the single most important blood marker for cardiovascular risk. Unlike traditional cholesterol tests, ApoB measures the actual number of particles that can enter the arterial wall. LDL-C tells you how much cholesterol is present; ApoB tells you how many particles are carrying it. And it is the particles that drive risk.

MTHFR is a genetic variant that affects methylation, detoxification, and how your body uses folate and B vitamins. Social media has turned it into a buzzword and a source of unnecessary fear. The truth is simpler: MTHFR is not a diagnosis and not a destiny. It simply means your body may need more support in certain pathways. It is a map, not a sentence. Understanding it alongside homocysteine and ApoB gives you a far more complete picture of your long-term health.

* * *

Sleep, Stress, and the Metrics That Matter

Sleep is not rest. Sleep is repair. Your sleep cycles determine hormone production, metabolic stability, memory consolidation, emotional regulation, inflammation control, cellular repair, and nervous system balance. Tracking sleep is not about perfection. It is about awareness. When you monitor REM, deep sleep, heart rate variability, resting heart rate, sleep latency, and sleep interruptions, you learn how your body is coping with life and what conditions help you heal.

Heart rate variability, or HRV, deserves its own moment of attention. HRV measures the tiny variations in time between each heartbeat, and it is one of the most accurate real-time indicators of nervous system health available without a clinical visit. A higher HRV generally signals that your nervous system is flexible, adaptive, and resilient. A suppressed HRV signals stress, overtraining, poor recovery, or sympathetic overdrive. Tracking it regularly gives you a window into your body's actual readiness to heal, perform, and recover.

VO_2 max — the measurement of how efficiently your body uses oxygen — is one of the strongest predictors of longevity, cardiovascular health, metabolic resilience, mitochondrial efficiency, and aging rate. Elite longevity researchers call it the biological age score. Tracking VO_2 max is not about athleticism. It is about cellular youth. Alongside inflammation markers like hs-CRP, ferritin, fasting insulin, and liver enzymes, it gives you a comprehensive view of whether your body is in healing mode, survival mode, or overload mode. Inflammation is not destiny. It is a signal. And signals can be changed.

Your DNA is not your destiny. Your data is your direction. Your habits are your power.

CHAPTER FIFTEEN

YOU CAN'T MASTER WHAT YOU DON'T MEASURE – YOUR CALL TO ACTION

There is a moment in every healing journey when information is no longer enough. A moment when awareness must turn into action. A moment when a person — woman or man — decides that their health is no longer optional. It is a priority. This chapter is that moment.

The truth is this: you do not need to overhaul your entire life to take control of your health. You do not need perfection, discipline, or a thirty-step plan. You need clarity, courage, and one small step taken with intention. The future of medicine is collaborative. But the future of your health begins with you.

What You Can Do This Week

You do not need a full protocol to begin. You need momentum. Start by tracking one thing — not everything. Most people fail because they try to monitor everything at once: calories, macros, steps, sleep, water, supplements, mood, workouts, glucose, and more. That is not empowerment; that is overwhelm. This week, choose one metric that matters most to you: sleep hours, daily protein intake, steps, water, stress triggers, energy levels, meal timing. Tracking one thing builds awareness, and awareness builds change.

Add one supportive habit, and resist the urge to begin with restriction. People love to start with elimination — cut sugar, cut carbs, cut alcohol. But restriction triggers rebellion. Instead, add: a morning protein-rich breakfast, a ten-minute walk after meals, a consistent bedtime, a hydration goal, a five-minute breathing practice, or a daily sunlight exposure routine. When you add nourishment, your body naturally begins to release what no longer serves it.

Schedule one appointment you have been avoiding. Everyone has that appointment — the hormone panel, the metabolic check, the skin exam, the sleep evaluation, the primary care follow-up — that keeps getting pushed to later. Avoidance is a form of self-abandonment. Scheduling the appointment is an act of self-leadership. Clean up one corner of your environment this week, and write down your top three symptoms or goals. Those three items become your compass and your conversation starter with any provider.

* * *

The Questions Every Patient Should Ask

Empowered patients get better care — not because they are demanding, but because they are informed. Ask your provider what the root cause of your symptom is. If they cannot answer this, they are treating the surface, not the system. Ask whether there are lifestyle, hormonal, metabolic, or inflammatory factors contributing to what you are experiencing. This signals that you understand health is interconnected. Ask to look at trends over time instead of single lab values. One lab result is a snapshot; trends tell the story.

Ask for your full menu of options — both conventional and integrative. Ask what you can do between appointments to support your progress. Ask for a plan that reflects your biology, not a generic template. And ask what labs or assessments would give the clearest picture of what is happening in your body. These questions shift you from passive to active, from recipient to participant. They are the difference between being a patient and being the CEO of your own health.

* * *

How to Advocate for Yourself Starting Now

Advocacy is not confrontation. It is collaboration. Bring notes to every appointment — your top symptoms, your goals, any changes since your last visit, the questions you want answered. Speak in patterns, not isolated moments. Instead of saying

"I'm tired," say "I have been experiencing afternoon energy crashes for the last three months, especially after meals." Patterns help providers identify root causes. Use the phrase "I don't feel like myself." It is one of the most powerful sentences in medicine. It signals that something deeper is happening, even if labs look normal.

Ask for explanations, not assumptions. If something does not make sense, ask: Can you walk me through the reasoning behind this plan? Can you show me how this lab connects to my symptoms? You deserve understanding, not confusion. And remember, you are the expert on your body. Providers are experts in medicine. But you are the expert in your lived experience. Your intuition matters. Your symptoms matter. Your story matters. If you do not feel heard, seek a second perspective — not because your provider is wrong, but because you deserve partnership.

You are not "difficult" for wanting answers. You are not "dramatic" for wanting to feel better. You are not "high-maintenance" for wanting personalized care. You are advocating for the only body you will ever have. And that is not too much. That is leadership.

* * *

Your Health Is a Relationship, Not a Task

Your health is not a project. It is a relationship — with your body, your habits, your environment, your stress, your sleep, your hormones, your metabolism, your nervous system, and your future self. Healthy relationships require attention, compassion, and consistency, not perfection.

Here is your simple, powerful, actionable plan for this week: track one thing, add one supportive habit, schedule one appointment, upgrade one corner of your environment, and write down your top three symptoms or goals. Five steps. Five minutes of intention. Massive momentum. Because the truth is this: you do not need a new life to feel better. You need a new direction. And today, you choose that direction.

CHAPTER SIXTEEN

YOUR PERSONAL ROADMAP - A READER'S WORKBOOK

This section is designed to help you move from awareness to action. You do not need perfection. You do not need a full plan. You need clarity, honesty, and one small step at a time. Use these prompts as your personal guide — a place to think, reflect, and commit.

* * *

Section 1: Your Starting Point

How do you feel in your body right now?

Write freely. There is no right or wrong answer. What feels off? What feels good? What feels confusing? What feels like it needs the most attention?

Your reflection:

____

____

____

What are the top three symptoms or concerns you want to address?

These become your compass.

1. ______________________________________

2. ______________________________________

3. ______________________________________

What are the top three goals you want to achieve?

Think about energy, mood, strength, clarity, sleep, confidence, longevity. These become your direction.

1. ____

2. ____

3. ____

* * *

Section 2: Your One-Week Action Plan

I will track this one metric this week:

Sleep / Steps / Protein intake / Water / Stress triggers / Energy levels / Mood / Meal timing

I will track: ____

I will add this one supportive habit:

Morning protein breakfast / Walk after meals / Consistent bedtime / Hydration goal / 5-minute breathing practice / Daily sunlight

I will add: ____

The appointment I will schedule:

Appointment:

____

I will schedule it by:

____

The corner of my environment I will upgrade:

Pantry / Supplement drawer / Sleep environment / Workspace / Nighttime routine

I will upgrade:

____

* * *

Section 3: Advocate for Yourself

What patterns have you noticed in your symptoms?

Think about timing, triggers, cycles, meals, stress, sleep.

____

____

Questions I want to ask my provider at my next appointment:

1. ______________________________________

2. ______________________________________

3. ______________________________________

* * *

Section 4: Your Empowerment Statement

Complete the sentence below. This becomes your anchor — your reminder of why you are doing this.

"I am taking control of my health by:

____"

"This matters to me because:

____"

* * *

Section 5: Your Next 30 Days

Choose one focus area for the next month: Nervous system regulation / Metabolic recalibration / Hormonal harmony / Inflammation reduction / Personalized protocols

My 30-day focus:

____

Week 1:

Week 2:

Week 3:

Week 4:

---

* * *

Section 6: Your Future Self

Imagine yourself ninety days from now — clearer, stronger, more energized, more aligned. How do you want to feel? What will be different? What will you thank yourself for starting today?

____

____

____

____

____

____

CLOSING

YOU ARE NOT YOUR TEN YEAR OLD SELF, SO STOP LISTENING TO THEM

You are not your ten-year old self. There is a younger version of you who still lives inside your mind. A version somewhere between the ages of seven and twelve. A version who learned to survive long before they ever learned to thrive. A version who did not have language for their feelings, did not have control over their environment, and did not have the tools to understand their body or their needs.

Ten is often when we first learned to shrink ourselves. To doubt ourselves. To stay quiet, stay small, stay agreeable, stay invisible. Ten is often when we first learned that our needs might be "too much," our feelings might be "inconvenient," and our voice might be unwelcome. But here is the truth you need to hear — the truth that will change everything:

You are not ten years old anymore. Stop listening to them.

You are not that child. You are not that scared, confused, overwhelmed version of yourself who was just trying to make sense of the world. You are an adult with wisdom, experience, resilience, and strength. You have lived through things your ten-year-old self could never have imagined. You have survived storms that version of you would have collapsed under. You have built a life your ten-year-old self did not even know was possible.

So why are you still letting that version of you make decisions about your health, your confidence, your boundaries, your worth, and your future? Why are you still listening to the voice that says: "I don't want to bother anyone." "I don't want to be wrong." "I don't know enough." "I'm scared to ask." That voice is not your truth. That voice is your past. And your past does not get to run your future. Not anymore.

You have tools now. You have knowledge now. You have support now. You have a framework now — The Carrera Method™, a roadmap your ten-year-old self never had access to. You understand your nervous system. You understand your metabolism. You understand your hormones. You understand inflammation. You understand your patterns and your triggers and your needs.

It is time to stop letting childhood fear make adult decisions. It is time to stop letting old wounds shape new choices. It is time to stop letting the child you once were dictate the life you are trying to build. You are not fragile. You are not helpless. You are not behind. You are not broken. You are not too late. You are not too old. You are not too far gone. You are becoming. You are evolving. You are rising. You are remembering who you are — and who you were always meant to be.

And here is the most important part: you do not have to do it alone. You have a partner in this journey. A guide. A clinician who believes in you. A provider who sees your potential even when you forget it. Someone who stands beside you, not above you. Someone who empowers you, not lectures you. Someone who collaborates with you, not controls you.

You are Strong. Capable. Worthy. Resilient. Intelligent. Powerful. Whole.

This is your moment to step into your adult self — the self who knows better, chooses better, and leads with confidence. This is your moment to say: I am done living from old wounds. I am done shrinking to fit old stories. I am done letting fear make decisions. I am done abandoning myself. This is your moment to choose your health. Your strength. Your clarity. Your energy. Your boundaries. Your voice. Your future.

You are not the version of you who did not know how to ask for help. You are not the version who did not understand your body. You are the adult who gets to rewrite the story. You are the adult who gets to choose healing. You are the adult who gets to choose empowerment. You are the adult who gets to choose yourself.

And you deserve to choose yourself — fully, boldly, unapologetically.

So take a breath. Stand tall. Lift your chin. Place your hand on your heart. And remind yourself:

"I am not who I used to be. I am who I decide to become."

Your younger self survived. Your current self will thrive. Your future self will thank you. And every step of the way, Carrera Telehealth and Wellness is right here with you.

Common Misconceptions About Your Health - Corrected

MYTH VS. TRUTH

Decades of misinformation, rushed appointments, and one-size-fits-all medicine have left most people carrying a set of beliefs about their health that are simply not true. The following myths are ones I encounter in my practice every single week. Read them carefully. See which ones you have believed. Then let the truth replace them.

MYTH #1

"My labs came back normal, so I must be healthy."

TRUTH

Normal lab values are based on population averages — and the average American is overweight, inflamed, and metabolically compromised. "Normal" means you fall within the range of what is common, not what is optimal. The markers that predict long-term health outcomes — ApoB, fasting insulin, homocysteine, high-sensitivity C-reactive protein, waist-to-height ratio — are rarely included in a standard panel. You can have entirely "normal" results and still be years into a trajectory toward heart disease, type 2 diabetes, or hormonal collapse. Normal is not a destination. It is a warning that you are keeping pace with a sick population.

MYTH #2

"Fatigue, brain fog, and weight gain are just part of getting older."

TRUTH

They are common with age — but common is not the same as inevitable. These symptoms are nearly always signs of an addressable underlying issue: hormonal imbalance, mitochondrial dysfunction, thyroid inefficiency, chronic low-grade inflammation, disrupted sleep architecture, or metabolic dysregulation. Age does not cause these conditions. Years of unaddressed stress, poor sleep, nutrient depletion, and a dysregulated nervous system do. Every one of those factors is modifiable. The body does not have an expiration date on healing — it has a threshold for how long it will wait for you to start listening.

MYTH #3

"If something were really wrong, my doctor would have caught it."

TRUTH

Your doctor is working inside a system that allocates eleven minutes per visit, reimburses for reactive care, and has no structural incentive to investigate what is not yet a diagnosable disease. This is not an indictment of individual physicians — most are skilled, caring, and doing their best within a broken infrastructure. It is an indictment of the system itself. Dysfunction accumulates for years before it crosses the threshold into a billable diagnosis. By the time it does, intervention is far more expensive, far more complex, and far less reversible. The system was built to catch you when you fall — not to prevent the fall.

MYTH #4

“Hormone therapy is dangerous and only for women in menopause.”

TRUTH

The fear around hormone therapy largely traces back to a single, widely misreported study from 2002 that has since been substantially re-analyzed and recontextualized. When prescribed appropriately, in the right form, at the right dose, and at the right time in a person’s hormonal trajectory, hormone optimization is one of the most evidence-supported tools available for protecting cardiovascular health, bone density, cognitive function, metabolic stability, and quality of life. It is not exclusively a women’s issue. Men experience progressive testosterone decline beginning in their thirties, with profound effects on energy, body composition, mood, libido, and longevity. Hormonal optimization is not about defying aging. It is about aging with your biology, not against it.

MYTH #5

"Peptides are experimental and unsafe — only bodybuilders use them."

TRUTH

Peptides are biological signaling molecules — your body makes them naturally, and has been using them to regulate healing, metabolism, immune function, and cellular repair your entire life. The GLP-1 medications that have transformed metabolic medicine globally are peptides. The FDA-approved drugs Trulicity, Ozempic, Mounjaro, and Wegovy are all peptide-based therapies. The emerging regenerative peptides used in personalized medicine — BPC-157, TB-500, CJC-1295, and others — have extensive preclinical literature and growing clinical application. Like any medical tool, they require appropriate clinical supervision, proper sourcing, and individualized dosing. The problem is not peptides. The problem is peptides obtained from unregulated sources and used without medical oversight.

MYTH #6

"I just need to eat less and exercise more."

TRUTH

If this advice worked, the nation would not be in the metabolic crisis it is in. Persistent weight gain and resistance to loss are rarely simply a matter of willpower or effort. They are almost always the downstream result of hormonal dysregulation, insulin resistance, chronic cortisol elevation, disrupted sleep, mitochondrial inefficiency, or a combination of several. Telling a metabolically dysregulated person to eat less and move more is the clinical equivalent of telling someone with a broken leg to walk it off. The instruction is not wrong in principle — it is profoundly insufficient in practice. The body's metabolic set point must be addressed before behavioral changes can produce and sustain the results people are working for.

MYTH #7

"Wellness is a luxury I can't afford."

TRUTH

Chronic disease is the luxury you cannot afford. The average American with type 2 diabetes spends over $16,000 per year on healthcare. A single cardiac event can generate six figures in medical debt. The long-term cost of ignoring your metabolic and hormonal health — in dollars, in lost productivity, in quality of life, in years — dwarfs the cost of prevention by an order of magnitude. Investing in your health now is not an indulgence. It is the most financially rational decision you can make. Sick care is expensive. Proactive wellness is an investment that compounds.

MYTH #8

"I've tried everything. Nothing works for me."

TRUTH

You have not tried everything. You have tried a series of disconnected interventions — usually applied in the wrong order, on a foundation that was not prepared to receive them. You tried the diet before your nervous system was regulated.

You tried the hormone therapy before your metabolism was supported. You tried the supplements before your inflammation was addressed. You tried the peptides before the gut was healed. The interventions may have been sound. The sequence was wrong. The Carrera Method™ is built specifically for the person who has "tried everything" — because the answer is rarely a new intervention. It is a new order.

Real Stories. Real Results. Real People.

PATIENT TRANSFORMATIONS

The following case studies represent the kind of transformation that becomes possible when The Carrera Method™ is applied in the right order, with the right tools, and with the full clinical attention each patient deserves. Names and identifying details have been changed to protect patient privacy. The clinical details, lab values, and outcomes are real.

As you read these stories, notice what they have in common: not a single one of these patients was broken. Every one of them had been failed — by a system that normalized their symptoms, dismissed their instincts, and never looked closely enough to find what was happening. What changed was not the person. What changed was the approach.

Patient #1 - Ryan

"Working with Dr. Carrera and her team has been incredible. Zepbound has given me the consistency I needed, and her support from Carrera Telehealth and Wellness has made all the difference. I have seen amazing progress in strength and overall health, and adding NAD + therapy has further boosted my energy and recovery. I am grateful for the guidance and encouragement every step of the way. Excited to share my before and after with Carrera Telehealth and Wellness.

* * *

Patient #2 - Melissa

"I stopped looking in the mirror because I didn't recognize the woman staring back at me. My health had hit an all-time low. It was time for a change, but I needed more help than just going to the gym. I found Dr. Carrera, and she helped me recognize the woman in the mirror again and reclaim my life.

Insurance companies can be difficult to navigate, but she took that stress away as well and helped me get the medication I needed and deserved. If you're on the fence, take a leap of faith and just do it! No regrets."

* * *

Patient #3 - Marsha

"My lifestyle was very sedentary. I work from home and spend most of the day sitting. At 175 pounds, I felt uncomfortable in my body and was carrying more weight than was healthy for my 5'7" frame.

I was skeptical about trying semaglutide. Medications have always made me nervous, and with my lack of exercise, I doubted it would work for me anyway.

After talking with my cardiologist, I asked whether he thought I should give it a try. His response was an enthusiastic, '100% YES!' He gave me the all-clear to move forward, so I decided, 'What the heck? I'll try it.'

By the end of April, I was down to 145 pounds. The weight seemed to melt away—even though I still worked from home and spent most of the day sitting.

To support my health, I committed to drinking a daily protein shake and added collagen, fiber, and cottage cheese to increase my protein intake. I also made sure to eat nutritious meals, so I stayed properly nourished throughout the process.

One of the biggest surprises was that my heart palpitations improved dramatically.

Looking back, the only thing I wish I had done differently was join a gym sooner to maintain muscle mass. My next goal is to build strength, tone my body, and continue feeling healthier and stronger every day."

* * *

THRIVE ASSESSMENT

Where Are You on the Spectrum From Surviving to Thriving?

Answer each question honestly. This is not a diagnostic tool — it is a mirror. The goal is not a perfect score. The goal is clarity about where you are starting, so you know exactly where to begin.

For each statement, choose the response that most accurately reflects your experience over the past 30 days.

* * *

SECTION A: Energy & Sleep

---

1. I wake up feeling genuinely rested and ready for the day.

□ Never □ Rarely □ Sometimes □ Often □ Always

2. My energy is stable throughout the day without relying on caffeine or sugar.

□ Never □ Rarely □ Sometimes □ Often □ Always

3. I fall asleep easily and stay asleep through the night.

□ Never □ Rarely □ Sometimes □ Often □ Always

4. I recover quickly after physical or emotional exertion.

□ Never □ Rarely □ Sometimes □ Often □ Always

5. I have enough energy at the end of the day to be present with the people I love.

□ Never □ Rarely □ Sometimes □ Often □ Always

* * *

SECTION B: Mood & Mental Clarity

---

6. I feel emotionally regulated and resilient under stress.

□ Never □ Rarely □ Sometimes □ Often □ Always

7. My thinking is clear, focused, and sharp.

□ Never □ Rarely □ Sometimes □ Often □ Always

8. I feel like myself — not a depleted or diminished version of myself.

□ Never □ Rarely □ Sometimes □ Often □ Always

9. I am able to handle unexpected challenges without feeling overwhelmed.

□ Never □ Rarely □ Sometimes □ Often □ Always

10. I experience genuine moments of joy, creativity, and engagement.

□ Never □ Rarely □ Sometimes □ Often □ Always

* * *

SECTION C: Body & Metabolism

---

11. My weight is stable and responds appropriately when I make lifestyle changes.

□ Never □ Rarely □ Sometimes □ Often □ Always

12. I feel strong and capable in my body.

□ Never □ Rarely □ Sometimes □ Often □ Always

13. My digestion is comfortable and consistent.

□ Never □ Rarely □ Sometimes □ Often □ Always

14. I rarely experience bloating, inflammation, joint pain, or unexplained physical discomfort.

□ Never □ Rarely □ Sometimes □ Often □ Always

15. My hunger and cravings feel manageable and appropriate.

□ Never □ Rarely □ Sometimes □ Often □ Always

* * *

SECTION D: Hormones & Vitality

---

16. My libido feels appropriate for my age and life circumstances.

□ Never □ Rarely □ Sometimes □ Often □ Always

17. I do not experience significant hormonal fluctuations affecting my mood or body.

□ Never □ Rarely □ Sometimes □ Often □ Always

18. My skin, hair, and nails reflect a body that is well-nourished and healthy.

□ Never □ Rarely □ Sometimes □ Often □ Always

19. I feel vital and physically alive — not just functional.

□ Never □ Rarely □ Sometimes □ Often □ Always

20. I am aging in a way that feels aligned with how I live, not despite it.

□ Never □ Rarely □ Sometimes □ Often □ Always

* * *

SECTION E: Mindset & Self-Leadership

---

21. I take proactive steps to manage my health rather than waiting for problems to arise.

□ Never □ Rarely □ Sometimes □ Often □ Always

22. I advocate clearly for myself in medical settings.

□ Never □ Rarely □ Sometimes □ Often □ Always

23. I understand my key health numbers and what they mean.

□ Never □ Rarely □ Sometimes □ Often □ Always

24. I invest in my health — in time, attention, and resources — consistently.

□ Never □ Rarely □ Sometimes □ Often □ Always

25. I believe that thriving — not just surviving — is available to me.

□ Never □ Rarely □ Sometimes □ Often □ Always

Scoring Your Assessment

Never = 0 points | Rarely = 1 point | Sometimes = 2 points | Often = 3 points | Always = 4 points

My Total Score: ________ / 100

Where Are You on the Spectrum from Surviving to Thriving?

0 – 25: Survival Mode

Your body is doing its best under significant strain. The foundation needs attention before anything else can change. Begin with Pillar 1 — nervous system regulation — and work steadily from there. You are not behind. You are beginning.

26 – 50: Functioning But Depleted

You are managing — but you know something is missing. The gap between where you are and where you want to be is real and addressable. Pillars 1 and 2 will produce the fastest and most noticeable shift. You are closer than you think.

51 – 75: Building Momentum

You have made real progress in some areas and have a solid foundation to build on. The remaining gaps are specific and targetable. Focus on the sections where your scores were lowest — those are your highest-leverage opportunities.

76 – 100: Thriving

You are operating from a strong foundation of health. Continue investing in maintenance, monitoring, and optimization. Use this score as a baseline to return to every quarter to track your trajectory over time.

My lowest-scoring section: ______________________________

The one change I will make this week based on my score:

____

____

____

____

____

____

____

____

____

____

____

____

Quick Reference

The Carrera Method™ at-a-Glance

The 5 Pillars — In Order

---

1. NERVOUS SYSTEM REGULATION

The master regulator. Stabilize this first or nothing else holds. Tools: sleep optimization, breathwork, cortisol support, circadian rhythm anchoring, stress chemistry management.

2. METABOLIC RECALIBRATION

Fuel the system correctly. Tools: protein-forward nutrition, glucose stability, hydration, electrolytes, mitochondrial support, reduction of inflammatory dietary inputs.

3. HORMONAL HARMONY

Balance the body's chemical messengers. Tools: comprehensive hormone panel, targeted optimization of estrogen, progesterone, testosterone, thyroid, DHEA, cortisol, insulin.

4. INFLAMMATION REDUCTION & CELLULAR REPAIR

Calm the fire. Tools: gut healing, micronutrient repletion, mitochondrial repair, anti-inflammatory nutrition, environmental exposure reduction.

5. PERSONALIZED OPTIMIZATION

Layer in advanced tools once the foundation is solid. Tools: peptide therapies, regenerative protocols, genetic insights, longevity monitoring, telehealth-guided precision care.

* * *

The Lab Panel That Actually Tells the Truth

Ask your provider for these markers at your next visit. If they push back, find a provider who won't.

Metabolic & Cardiovascular

Fasting insulin • HbA1c • Fasting glucose • ApoB • Triglycerides • HDL • LDL • Homocysteine • hs-CRP • Waist-to-height ratio

Hormonal

Free & total testosterone • Estradiol • Progesterone • DHEA-S • TSH • Free T3 • Free T4 • Reverse T3 • Cortisol (AM) • Sex hormone binding globulin (SHBG)

Nutritional & Cellular

Vitamin D (25-OH) • Vitamin B12 • Ferritin • Iron & TIBC • Magnesium (RBC) • Zinc • Omega-3 index • MTHFR • Complete metabolic panel • CBC

Questions to Ask at Every Appointment

"What is the root cause of this symptom — not just the name for it?"

"Are there hormonal, metabolic, inflammatory, or nervous system factors contributing?"

"Can we look at trends over time rather than a single snapshot?"

"What are all my options, both conventional and integrative?"

"What can I do between appointments to support my progress?"

"Can we personalize this plan to my biology and goals?"

"I don't feel like myself. I need us to look deeper."

* * *

The 5-Step Weekly Practice

These five actions, done consistently, will produce measurable results within 30 days.

Monday — Measure

Check in with one biometric: sleep score, resting heart rate, HRV, or energy level on a scale of 1–10. Write it down.

Wednesday — Nourish

Ensure your protein intake hits your target. Add one anti-inflammatory food. Drink your water.

Friday — Regulate

Five minutes of intentional nervous system downregulation: box breathing, a slow walk, prayer, or stillness.

Sunday — Reflect

Three things your body did well this week. One thing you want to do differently next week.

Any Day — Advocate

Schedule the appointment you have been avoiding. Ask the question you have been afraid to ask. Take the action you have been deferring.

Notes — My Health Journey

Use this space to capture your thoughts, observations, questions for your provider, or anything this book brought to the surface.

Not the End, Just the Beginning... Let's THRIVE

In the words of my dear friend Leah, you don't just need a partner — you need the kind of support system where **1 + 1 doesn't equal 2... it equals 11**. The right partnership multiplies your strength, your clarity, and your capacity to thrive. The same is true in healthcare. Choosing the right provider and the right team determines your longevity, your confidence, and your ability to live a life that is truly *beyond better*.

At Carrera Telehealth & Wellness, my team and I walk beside you, not ahead of you — and with our expanded partnership with Dr. Stefano Sinicropi, MD, orthopedic spinal surgeon in **ABOVE GENETICS**, we now bring you an even broader spectrum of traditional, regenerative, and cutting-edge medical care. There is always room for you in our VIP community, where we empower you and your loved ones with the knowledge, tools, and emerging advancements that shape the future of regenerative medicine. I hope you enjoyed this book, and I look forward to creating that "11 partnership" with you — one that elevates your health, your vitality, and your entire life.

With Love and Care,

Dr. Danielle Carrera

ABOUT THE AUTHOR

Dr. Danielle Carrera DNP, APRN

Dr. Danielle Carrera is a Doctor of Nursing Practice and autonomous Advanced Practice Registered Nurse, trained at the University of South Florida and licensed across multiple states nationwide. She is the founder and CEO of Carrera Telehealth and Wellness, a modern medical practice built on her core belief that patients deserve more than the absence of illness — they deserve the opportunity to truly thrive.

Her clinical career spans to almost three decades and encompasses hospital medicine, urgent care, psychiatric care, long-term care and care management, government-sponsored prevention programs for first responders, underserved community health, women's health, hormone replacement for men and woman, aesthetics - wellness training and care, insurance-based managed care, national provider speaker for metabolic and endocrine disorders and regenerative medicine.

She has practiced in some of the most demanding and diverse healthcare environments in the country, which has given her a clinical perspective that is simultaneously broad and deeply practical.

Dr. Carrera served as a national provider speaker for Eli Lilly's GLP-1 and dual-agonist medications, including Trulicity and Mounjaro. She has been involved in pharmaceutical board advisory roles and has taught providers, nurses, and patients across the country about the evolving science of metabolic medicine, weight management, and peptide-based therapeutics.

She is the architect of The Carrera Method™, a five-pillar integrative framework for achieving optimal health through nervous system regulation, metabolic recalibration, hormonal harmony, inflammation reduction, and personalized optimization. The method reflects her core clinical philosophy: that the body is not the problem — it is the messenger — and that lasting health is not achieved through symptom suppression but through building the physiological conditions in which the body can genuinely thrive.

Dr. Carrera is based in the Tampa Bay area of Florida and cares for patients nationwide through Carrera Telehealth & Wellness. She has now expanded her reach to **ABOVE GENETICS**, partnering with Dr. Stefano Sinicropi, MD — an orthopedic spinal surgeon who shares her mission to empower every individual to become the CEO of their own health. Together, they bring a unified vision of advanced, integrative, and regenerative medicine to patients across the country, ensuring that each person has access to the highest level of expertise, innovation, and support on their journey to lifelong wellness.

Dr. Carrera is a mother of two, a wife, a competitive spirit and fitness guru, a woman who rebuilt herself more than once, a leader who refuses to settle for "average", a partner that will always tell you to hold steadfast and a living example of what it means to become the CEO of your own health.

CARRERA TELEHEALTH & WELLNESS

Carrera
TELEHEALTH & WELLNESS
VIRTUAL & TELEPHONIC MEDICAL SERVICES

PERSONALIZED HEALTHCARE & WELLNESS FROM THE CONVENIENCE OF YOUR HOME, OFFICE, COFFEE SHOP, VACATION, AND MORE...

SCAN ME

"ABOVE GENETICS" VIP COMMUNITY

Your DNA is not your destiny.

Your daily decisions are.

Precision genetic testing, mitochondrial analysis, and a clinician-led longevity community for high-performing individuals who want proactive, personalized control of their future health.

www.ingramcontent.com/pod-product-compliance
Lightning Source LLC
LaVergne TN
LVHW052319200926
848481LV00002B/603

* 9 7 9 8 9 9 3 9 5 1 7 2 0 *